CYTOKINES AND CYTOKINE RECEPTORS

Titles published in the series:

*Antigen-presenting Cells
*Complement
*Cytokines and Cytokine Receptors
DNA Replication
Enzyme Kinetics
Gene Structure and Transcription 2nd edn
Genetic Engineering
*Immune Recognition
*B Lymphocytes
*Lymphokines
Membrane Structure and Function
Molecular Basis of Inherited Disease 2nd edn
Molecular Genetic Ecology
Protein Biosynthesis
Protein Engineering
Protein Structure
Protein Targeting and Secretion
Regulation of Enzyme Activity
*The Thymus

*Published in association with the British Society for Immunology.

Series editors

David Rickwood

Department of Biology, University of Essex, Wivenhoe Park,
Colchester, Essex CO4 3SQ, UK

David Male

Institute of Psychiatry, De Crespigny Park, Denmark Hill,
London SE5 8AF, UK

CYTOKINES AND CYTOKINE RECEPTORS

Anne S. Hamblin

Senior Lecturer in Immunology, Department of Pathology and
Infectious Diseases, The Royal Veterinary College,
Royal College Street, London NW1 0TU, UK

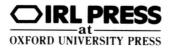

⬡IRL PRESS
──── at ────
OXFORD UNIVERSITY PRESS

Oxford University Press, Walton Street, Oxford OX2 6DP

Oxford   New York   Toronto
Delhi   Bombay   Calcutta   Madras   Karachi
Kuala Lumpur   Singapore   Hong Kong   Tokyo
Nairobi   Dar es Salaam   Cape Town
Melbourne   Auckland   Madrid
and associated companies in
Berlin   Ibadan

Oxford is a trade mark of Oxford University Press

In Focus is a registered trade mark of the Chancellor, Masters, and Scholars
of the University of Oxford trading as Oxford University Press

Published in the United States
by Oxford University Press Inc., New York

A catalogue record for this book is available from the British Library

Library of Congress Cataloging in Publication Data
Hamblin, Anne S.
Cytokines and cytokine receptors/by Anne S. Hamblin.
(In focus)
Includes bibliographical references and index.
1. Cytokines.   2. Cytokines–Receptors.   I. Title.   II. Series:
In focus (Oxford, England)
[DNLM: 1. Cytokines–metabolism.   2. Receptors, Immunologic.   QW
568 H199c 1993]
QR185.8.C95H35   1993   616.07'9–dc20   93–1761

ISBN 0–19–963388–6

Typeset by Footnote Graphics, Warminster, Wiltshire
Printed by Interprint Ltd., Malta

Preface

Cytokines are a group of signalling molecules involved in communication between cells, including those of the immune system. Cytokine-mediated events occur during the initiation and effector stages of immune responses and the development of haematopoietic cells. Consequently, an understanding of cytokine biology is essential to understand how immune reactions develop and how they are controlled. Recent work has, however, shown how important cytokines are in other physiological responses of the body.

For many years the identity and characteristics of individual cytokines were obscured by the difficulty in purifying them and the minute quantities which were active in biological assays. Within the last 5 years there has been an explosion of information on cytokine and cytokine receptor structures and genes, along with a clarification of the roles of individual cytokines. This was a consequence of developments in molecular biology, which has produced gene clones encoding many of these molecules.

This book focuses particularly on the structures and functions of the best characterized cytokines, and it brings together detailed information from many primary sources. The growing evidence that cytokines are involved in the immunopathology of a number of diseases, and may provide new therapeutic modalities, provides the incentive for combined extensive investigation of these molecules.

A. S. Hamblin

Acknowledgements

I would like to thank the many immunological colleagues who provided advice and information during the writing of this book. I would like to thank Ms Dora Paterson for typing the monograph. Particular thanks go to my husband and children for their support; I would like to dedicate this monograph to them.

Contents

Abbreviations

ADCC	antibody-dependent cell-mediated cytotoxicity
AIDS	acquired immune deficiency syndrome
anti-Tac	anti-IL2 receptor (P55 or α chain) antibody
APC	antigen-presenting cell
BCG	Bacillus Calmette-Guérin
BCGF	B cell growth factor
BFU	blast forming unit
CD	cluster of differentiation
cDNA	complementary deoxyribonucleic acid
CFU	colony forming unit
CFU-E	CFU erythrocyte
CFU-Eo	CFU eosinophil
CFU-GEMM	CFU granulocyte, erythrocyte, monocyte, megakaryocyte
CFU-GM	CFU granulocyte, macrophage
CFU-Meg	CFU megakaryocyte
CR1	complement receptor 1
CSF	colony stimulating factor
E	erythropoietin
ELAM	endothelial leucocyte adhesion molecule
ELISA	enzyme-linked immunosorbent assay
f-Met-Leu-Phe	formyl-methionyl leucyl phenylalanine
G-CSF	granulocyte-CSF
GM-CSF	granulocyte-macrophage-CSF
HIV	human immunodeficiency virus
HTLV	human T cell leukaemia virus
ICAM	intercellular adhesion molecule
IRMA	immunoradiometric assay
IFN	interferon
Ig	immunoglobulin
IL	interleukin
kDa	kilodalton
LAK	lymphokine activated killer cell
LIF	leukaemia inhibitory factor
LPS	lipopolysaccharide

LT	lymphotoxin
MCAF	macrophage chemotactic and activating factor
M-CSF	macrophage-CSF
MHC	major histocompatibility complex
mRNA	messenger ribonucleic acid
NK	natural killer
PAGE	poly acrylamide gel electrophoresis
PKC	protein kinase C
PMA	phorbol myristate acetate
R	receptor
RIA	radioimmunoassay
SAC	*Staphylococcus aureus* Cowan strain 1
SDS	sodium dodecyl sulphate
T_C	cytotoxic T cells
TGF	transforming growth factor
TFR	transferrin receptor
T_H	helper T cells
TNF	tumour necrosis factor

1

Cytokines

Discovery

The 1960s were a time of intense investigation into the origins and regulation of cellular immune responses. At that time, cell-mediated immunity to antigens was assessed *in vivo* by the production and cellular transfer of delayed-type hypersensitivity skin reactions, and *in vitro* by the transformation of sensitized lymphocytes by specific antigen and the inhibition of macrophage migration following interaction between lymphoid populations containing macrophages, sensitized lymphocytes, and specific antigen. The demonstration that cell-free soluble factors generated *in vitro* in the culture supernatants of sensitized lymphocytes incubated with antigen, (i) could produce skin lesions similar to delayed-type hypersensitivity (1), (ii) were mitogenic for lymphocytes (2), and (iii) could cause macrophage migration inhibition (3), suggested that molecular mediators were involved in cellular immune responses (*Figure 1.1*).

To interpret these findings, the term lymphokine was introduced in 1969 to describe 'cell-free soluble factors generated by the interaction of sensitized lymphocytes with specific antigen and expressed without reference to the immunological specificity' (4). The generic term was chosen to emphasize their origins (lymphocytes) and also their role in the maintenance of the physiology of the immune system (kinesis). The evidence implicated thymus-derived T lymphocytes as the cells which interacted specifically with antigen to release the lymphokines which then acted non-specifically on target cells. Further work showed that crude culture supernatants could influence the *in vitro* behaviour of a large number of target cells in many different ways, and led to the view that many cellular immune interactions were regulated by soluble factors (5).

During the 1970s the term lymphokine became more widely used, to describe not only the large number of biological activities of antigen-activated T lymphocytes presumed, but not proven, to be ascribable to biochemical factors in the culture supernatants, but also those in culture supernatants of lymphocytes non-specifically activated with mitogens (e.g. phytohaemagglutinin and concanavalin A) or cultured cell lines of both lymphoid and non-lymphoid origin. Similar

1

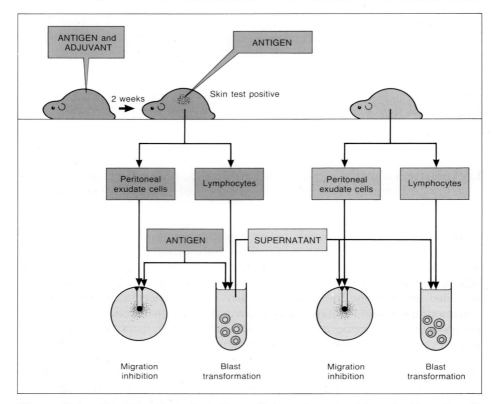

Figure 1.1.   Demonstration of cytokines. Guinea pigs were injected with antigen in complete Freund's adjuvant: after 2 weeks the animals gave a positive delayed hyper-sensitivity skin test to the antigen, their peritoneal exudate cells showed inhibited migration in the presence of antigen and their lymphocytes proliferated in response to antigen. These effects could be reproduced on cells from untreated guinea pigs, using tissue culture supernatants of antigen-activated lymphocytes from the immunized animals.

activities were also found in body fluids such as serum and urine. During this period there was considerable scepticism regarding the role and even existence of distinct soluble factors regulating the immune system. For many workers, the large number of activities [more than 100 were cited in a list published in 1979 (5)], their disparate sources, and their lack of biochemical characterization were enough to suggest that the whole concept was based on artefact.

However, by the late 1970s, a number of technical advances had led to the purification to homogeneity of some of the factors. This progress has continued with the introduction of molecular biology techniques, resulting in a description of the structure of these mediators and a better understanding of their function.

It is now clear that cells of the immune system secrete and respond to soluble factors which exert wide-ranging effects. Whilst T cells and macrophages are a major source, other cells can also produce them. The factors are important not only in the regulation and differentiation of cells responding to antigen, but also in the inflammatory and physiological interactions between immune and non-immune cells.

Nomenclature and classification

At first, the factors were named on the basis of the activity they produced *in vivo*, or more frequently *in vitro*. Their names were abbreviated to acronyms. For example, migration inhibition factor, or MIF, was generated in cultures of antigen-activated lymphocytes and, when added to non-immune peritoneal macrophages, inhibited their migration from capillary tubes (3,5).

Various terms have been introduced in attempts to order the enormous number of acronyms and titles applied to substances secreted by cells. Thus 'monokine' and 'cytokine' were used to denote the fact that monocytes were the source of some biological mediators and that non-lymphoid cells produced others, and to differentiate them from lymphokines produced by lymphocytes (6). The term interleukin (between leucocytes) first appeared in 1979 to 'free nomenclature from the constraints associated with definitions by single bio-assays' (7). Constraining bioassay-based names were felt to be inappropriate when it became clear that a variety of biological activities were actually different effects of the same substance. For example, the factor derived from monocytes causing lymphocyte activation, which had previously been known as lymphocyte activating factor (LAF) appeared the same as that previously known as mitogenic protein (MP), T cell-replacing factor III (TRF-III), B cell activating factor (BAF) and a B cell differentiation factor (BDF). The factor was renamed inter-leukin 1 (IL-1). At the same time it was realized that T cell growth factor (TCGF) was the same as thymocyte mitogenic factor (TMF) and this was renamed IL-2 (7). The terms interleukin, lymphokine, monokine, and cytokine are still used widely, but the term cytokine has emerged as an umbrella term to describe this group of soluble proteins which influence cells of the immune system.

The attribution of a variety of biological effects to the same substance, as described above for IL-1 and IL-2, was made possible by improved biochemical analysis of cell supernatants allowing purification of factors to homogeneity and then production of large amounts by genetic engineering. Currently, the cyto-kines include 10 interleukins which are recognized by the Nomenclature of the International Union of Immunological Societies (IUIS) Committee (8) as well as a number of other cytokines which retain their activity-based names (*Table 1.1*). Other interleukins have been described, e.g. IL-11, IL-12, and IL-13, but have not yet been officially recognized. It should be emphasized that the name of a cytokine may not be a very good guide to its properties. Thus interferon γ (IFN-γ) is more of interest for its ability to activate macrophages and other cells than for its antiviral activity and tumour necrosis factor (TNF) is more important for its inflammatory activity than for causing tumour necrosis.

Table 1.1   Cloned cytokines and their alternative names

	Acronym	Alternative title
Interferons (α, β, and γ)	IFN-α,-β or -γ	
Interleukin 1α	IL-1α	Lymphocyte activating factor
Interleukin 1β	IL-1β	(LAF); mitogenic protein (MP); T cell replacing factor III (TRF-III); B cell activating factor (BAF); B cell differentiation factor (BDF); endogenous pyrogen (EP); leucocyte endogenous mediator (LEM); serum amyloid A (SAA) inducer; proteolysis inducing factor (PIF); catabolin; haematopoietin 1 (HP1); mononuclear cell factor (MCF)
Interleukin 2	IL-2	T cell growth factor (TCGF); thymocyte mitogenic factor (TMF)
Interleukin 3	IL-3	Multi-potential colony stimulating factor (multi-CSF); burst promoting activity (BP); haemapoietic cell growth factor (HPGF); persisting cell stimulating factor (PSF); mast cell growth factor (MCGF); haematopoietin 2 (HP2)
Interleukin 4	IL-4	B cell stimulating factor (BSF-1); T cell growth factor II (TCGF-II); mast cell growth factor II (MCGF-II); B cell growth factor I (BCGF-I);
Interleukin 5	IL-5	T cell replacing factor (TRF); B cell growth factor II (BCGF-II); eosinophil differentiation factor (EDF); IgA enhancing factor
Interleukin 6	IL-6	Interferon β_2 (IFN-β_2); B cell stimulation factor 2 (BSF-2); B cell differentiation factor (BCDF); hybridoma/plasmacytoma growth factor (HPGF); hepatocyte stimulating factor (HSF)
Interleukin 7	IL-7	Pre-B cell growth factor; lymphopoietin-1
Interleukin 8	IL-8	Monocyte-derived neutrophil chemotactic factor (MDNCF); neutrophil activating protein (NAP)
Interleukin 9	IL-9	p40; mast cell growth factor (MCGF); T-cell growth factor (TGF)
Interleukin 10	IL-10	Cytokine synthesis inhibiting factor (CSIF); B-cell derived thymocyte growth factor (B-TCGF); mast cell growth factor III (MCGF III)

Table 1.1 (*continued*)

	Acronym	Alternative title
Interleukin 11	IL-11	Interleukin 11
Interleukin 12	IL-12	Cytotoxic lymphocyte maturation factor (CLMF); natural killer cell stimulating factor (NKSF)
Granulocyte–macrophage colony stimulating factor	GM-CSF	Colony stimulating factor α (CSF-α); colony stimulating factor 2 (CSF-2)
Macrophage colony stimulating factor	M-CSF	Colony stimulating factor 1 (CSF-1)
Granulocyte colony stimulating factor	G-CSF	Colony stimulating factor β (CSF-β)
Tumour necrosis factor	TNF	Cachectin; tumour necrosis factor α (TNF-α)
Lymphotoxin	LT	Tumour necrosis factor β (TNF-β)

Whilst there is every reason to believe that many of the 100 activities described in 1979 are caused by the same factors, the actual number of cytokines remains to be determined. In this book the emphasis is on the structure and biological activity of some of those cytokines which have been cloned and which influence cells of the immune system. There are certainly other important cytokines which have yet to be cloned, and there are several cytokines which have been cloned which so far seem only to play minor roles in immunity. The extent of this book does not permit full description of these and the reader is referred to the general reading list for further information.

General aspects of cytokine structures and genetics

Early studies indicated that cytokines were proteins or glycoproteins which were not immunoglobulins. In spite of many attempts, further consistent biochemical analysis proved more difficult. In the first place, only small amounts of cytokines are made by cells in culture and therefore large cultures were needed to provide sufficient starting material for analysis. In the second place, activity was frequently lost on purification. Where information was acquired, it was often conflicting, particularly with respect to molecular size (9). Several technological advances provided better means to investigate the biochemical structure of cytokines. Cell lines and hybridomas could be grown in large volumes of culture medium from which the cytokine could be purified. The cells could often be stimulated with a cocktail of agents to superinduce production. By both these means, the amount of starting material for purification could be increased. As biochemical separation and detection methods for proteins became more sensitive, it became possible to purify cytokines to homogeneity from native sources

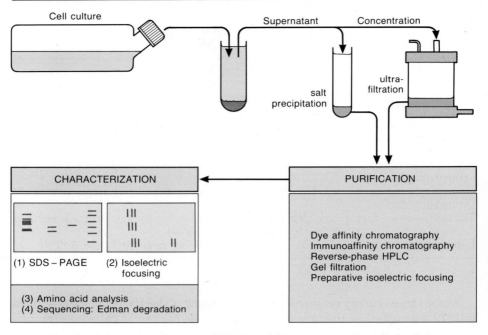

Figure 1.2.   Purification and characterization of cytokines from natural sources. The supernatant of a cell line producing the cytokine is obtained and the protein concentrated by salt precipitation or ultrafiltration. The cytokine is purified by successive fractionation methods, and the active fraction identified by immunoassay or bioassay at each stage. Analytical gels are used to characterize the purified cytokine.

(*Figure 1.2*). The amino acid composition and sequence of the homogeneous material could then be determined.

Large-scale production of cytokines is now usually by recombinant DNA methods. With the advent of gene cloning, the means to produce very large amounts of protein in prokaryotes or eukaryotes were established. The availability of large amounts of homogeneous protein has permitted better analysis of cytokine biological activity *in vivo* and *in vitro*, and has provided potential therapeutic agents for clinical trial. For cloning, the relevant gene is inserted into prokaryotes, such as *Escherichia coli*, or eukaryotes, such as yeast, which replicate rapidly. Since these sources can provide many thousand times the amount obtainable by conventional means and can be cultured continuously, they provide an excellent source of cytokines. The cytokine is often the major protein produced and its separation from vector proteins and contaminants is relatively straightforward.

Several approaches have been exploited to isolate cytokine gene sequences for cloning from cDNA libraries [*Figure 1.3* (9,10)]. In the first, oligonucleotides are prepared to match a portion of the amino acid sequence of the protein and these are used to probe cDNA libraries. This requires purification and partial sequencing of the protein by the methods described above. In the second and

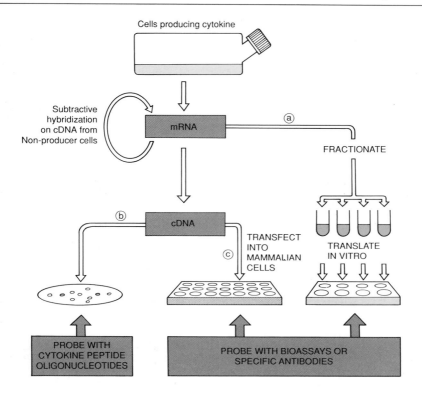

Figure 1.3. Strategies for identifying cytokines and their receptors. mRNA is isolated from cells stimulated to produce the cytokine required, or expressing the receptor. The mRNA of interest may be enriched by subtractive hybridization using cDNA generated from mRNA of a non-producer cell. The mRNA may be fractionated and translated directly to identify the cytokine by bioassay, or with cytokine-specific antibodies (**a**). Alternatively cDNA can be generated. If this is expressed in prokaryotes (**b**) positive clones can be identified with oligonucleotide probes based on the protein sequence of the cytokine derived by conventional techniques. cDNA can also be amplified and transfected directly into mammalian cells for identification of the expressed proteins (**c**). This is most useful for detecting cytokine receptor genes.

now more common approach, protein sequencing is circumvented by isolation of mRNA from an appropriate cell and this is used to screen the cDNA library. The mRNA selected is then translated *in vitro* or in *Xenopus* oocytes, and the translation product is detected by bioassay or by binding to an antibody if one is available (*Figure 1.3*). A particular feature of cytokines which has been exploited in these studies is the fact that mRNA expression is usually induced by stimulation of cells. The mRNA of interest may therefore be identified by comparison and subtraction of that from uninduced cells (plus–minus or subtractive hybridization). More recently direct expression strategies in *in vivo* or *in vitro* systems have been used to isolate the genes for cytokines. Here the cDNA prepared from cellular RNA is inserted into a plasmid that is able to direct the expression of the protein in mammalian cells. The plasmids are amplified in *Escherichia coli* and tranfected into mammalian cells. Detection of the protein of interest is then by bioassay, antibodies, or autoradiography. Once a double-stranded cDNA has been prepared by a technique not based on direct expression cloning it can be inserted via a plasmid into bacteria, yeast, or mammalian cells which replicate producing large amounts of protein.

Cloned cytokine genes and proteins can be sequenced and investigated in various ways. Site-directed mutagenesis may be used to alter single amino acids so that they no longer glycosylate or form disulphide bridges. Alternatively, cytokine genes may be engineered into yeast or mammalian cells which will glycosylate proteins to produce a more 'natural' product. In these ways the biological importance of glycosylation and disulphide bonds can be studied. Synthetic or cDNAs are used to probe a human genomic library to determine the structure of the gene. The chromosomal location of the gene is determined by hybridization to DNA from somatic cell hybrids containing known sets of chromosomes from the species under investigation.

Cytokines are encoded by genes for which there is only one copy per haploid cell. In common with most eukaryotic genes, the cytokine genes (with the exception of IFN-α and IFN-β genes which lack introns) are segmented, being composed of exons which are complementary to sequences in the mature mRNA and which are separated by introns which are not found in the mRNA (*Figure 1.4*).

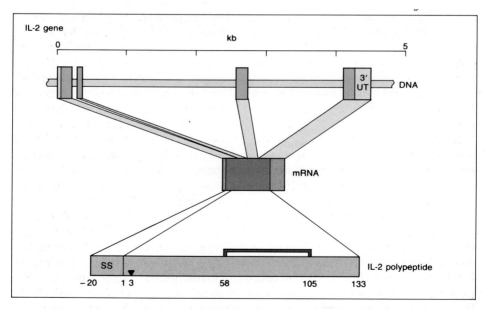

Figure 1.4.   Human IL-2 gene showing the gene structure of a typical cytokine. The IL-2 gene consists of four exons which generate a polypeptide of 155 amino acids. The first 20 residues are a signal sequence (SS) cleaved from the mature protein, and there is a disulphide link between cysteine residues at positions 58 and 105. The molecule is *O*-glycosylated at residue 3.

Most cytokine genes consist of three or four introns and four or five exons and are located on a number of different chromosomes (*Table 1.2*). It is of interest that in the human a number are located on the long arm of chromosome 5 and that TNF and lymphotoxin (LT) are closely linked on chromosome 6 within the major histocompatibility complex (MHC). The location of genes on the same chromosome raises the possibility that they may be closely linked and under the influence of common regulatory elements.

cDNAs for cytokines usually predict mature proteins of around 80–200 amino acids. Most have a clearly defined hydrophobic signal sequence of around 20 amino acids, which is cleaved to give the mature protein (*Figure 1.4*). It is notable that those factors derived from macrophages (TNF, IL-1α, and IL-1β) do not have such clearly defined signal sequences. Here a pre-sequence which is unusually long (70 or more amino acids) is cleaved from the mature protein. Since the signal sequences are associated with transport of the proteins out of the cell, this difference may represent an important difference in secretory mechanisms between macrophages and other cells.

Amino acid sequence data show that many cytokines contain cysteine residues which may be important in the formation of intramolecular disulphide bonds. Using site-directed mutagenesis and chemical reduction the importance of these disulphide bridges for the tertiary structure of the molecule and its biological activity has been determined for several of the cytokines.

Molecular weight determinations of cytokines purified from native sources frequently suggest that they are not homogeneous and that they are larger than predicted from the cloned genes. The discrepancies between predicted and observed molecular weights arise from post-translational modification, particularly glycosylation. Most cytokines are variably glycosylated (usually *N*-glycosylated) and the glycosylated proteins may form oligomers. Size estimations of natural proteins suggest a range of molecular weights which are reduced by separation under reducing conditions on SDS–PAGE. Further reductions in molecular weight heterogeneity may be achieved by incubation of the cytokine with glycosidases which cleave off glycosylated side chains. The function of the glycosylation is unclear since recombinant products made in *Escherichia coli*, which are not able to glycosylate proteins, often have the same biological activities. However, glycosylation may affect the half-life of cytokines *in vivo* and their distribution.

Cytokines are usually produced by cells in response to induction signals generated from the cell surface. The production of cytokines is strictly controlled at the level of transcription although this control process is incompletely understood. Regulatory elements are found in the DNA upstream from the coding DNA sequence which control initiation of transcription. Some cytokines, for example granulocyte–macrophage colony stimulating factor (GM-CSF), IL-2, IL-3, and IFN-γ, have common nucleotide sequences in the 5′ flanking region of their genes which may be important in the initiation of transcription and indeed in the coordinate expression of the genes so often seen on cell stimulation. Post-translational regulation affecting the stability of mRNAs also plays a role in controlling the production of some cytokines e.g. GM-CSF and G-CSF.

Table 1.2 Human cytokine structure

Cytokine	Native protein Mol. wt (kDa)	No. of amino acids		Glycosylation sites[c]	Cysteines	Genomic clone	
		Precursor	Mature protein			Intron/Exon	Location (chromosome)
IFN-α_1	16–27	189	166	None	4	None	9q13-q22
IFN-β	20	187	166	1(N)[c]	3	None	9q13
IFN-γ	20–24[a]	166	143	2(N)	2	3/4	12q24.1
IL-1α	17.5	271	159	None	None	6/7	2q12-q21
IL-1β	17.3	269	153	None	None	6/7	2q13-q21
IL-2	15–20	153	133	1(O)	3	4/5	4q26-q27
IL-3	14–30	152	133	2(N)	2	4/5	5q23-q31
IL-4	15–19	153	129	2(N)	6	3/4	5q23-q31
IL-5	22.5[a]	134	115	2(N)	2	3/4	5q23-q31
IL-6	26	212	184	2(N)	4	4/5	7q21-q14
IL-7	20–28	177	152	3(N)	6	5/6	8q12-q13
IL-8	8–10[a]	99	72	None	4	3/4	4q12-q21
IL-9	32–39	144	126	4(N)	10	4/5	5q31-32
IL-10	19[a]	178	160	1(N)	4		1
IL-11	23	199	180	None	0		
IL-12	Heterodimer of 35 and 40	253 and 328	197 and 306	3 and 4	7 and 10		
GM-CSF	22	144	127		4	3/4	5q21-5q32
G-CSF	18–22	204	174		5	4/5	17q21-q22
M-CSF	40–90[a]	554 or 256	522 or 224	10 or none	10 or 7	9/10	5q33.1
TNF	17[b]	233	157	None	2	3/4	6p21.3
LT	20–25	205	171	1(N)	0	3/4	6p21.3
TGF-β_1	12.5[a]	391	112	None	9		19q13.1

[a] Exists as homodimer; [b] exists as a trimer; [c] *N*- or *O*-glycosylation is indicated in parentheses.

Most molecular genetic studies on cytokines to date have been undertaken on mouse and human proteins with occasional information on other species. Comparison of both cDNA and genomic sequences of different cytokines in one species and the same cytokine between species has been used to determine possible relationships between cytokines as well as phylogenetic conservation of structure. Thus, IL-1α and IL-1β are structurally related and have the same or very similar biological activities, suggesting they may have arisen from gene duplication. IL-1α shows 61–65 per cent amino acid homology between human, rabbit, and mouse and IL-1β shows 27–33 per cent homology with IL-1α in the three species. These results suggest that the IL-1 genes arose from duplication before or during vertebrate evolution and then diverged independently. Homology between mouse and human cytokines ranges from close [e.g. IL-5 (67%)] to very poor [e.g. IL-3 (29%)] (11). Comparisons of the primary structures of different cytokines in one species have, however, generally not revealed related structures, with the exception of the chemokine family, which includes IL-8, which show conserved amino acid motifs (see Chapter 2).

Three-dimensional structures of a number of cytokines have now been determined from X-ray crystallography [12–15 (*Figure 1.5*)]. So far these structures show little similarity even when the biological activities are very similar, e.g. IL-1β and TNF. Some cytokines exist as polymers. Thus, whilst IL-1 and IL-2 exist as monomers TNF is found as a trimer and others, such as IL-8, M-CSF, and TGF-β, as dimers. By examination of these and other cytokine tertiary structures, predictions may be made regarding the parts of the molecule involved in binding to cytokine receptors. Information about the structure of receptors will allow molecular modelling of cytokine–receptor interactions.

General aspects of cytokine receptor structures and genetics

Cytokines are intercellular mediators which exert their effects through specific cell surface receptors. It is through understanding the interaction of cytokines with their receptors that we are beginning to see how the complex biology of cytokines may operate. Major advances have been made in the last few years in determining the structure of cytokine receptors. Three approaches have been used; direct expression cloning, purification of receptor molecules from cells that express them at high density, and subtractive hybridization. In contrast to the cytokines themselves, cytokine receptors do seem to form distinct families of cytokine structures (16). The three major families so far identified are, (i) those which are members of the immunoglobulin supergene family, (ii) those which have specifically conserved cysteine residues in the extracellular domain and a characteristic tryptophan-serine-x-tryptophan-serine (WSXWS) motif just proximal to the membrane spanning region (the haematopoietin receptor family) and, (iii) the TNF receptor family (*Figure 1.6*).

Most of these receptors are expressed at low density (100–1000 receptors per cell) although the numbers may increase when the cell is activated and may

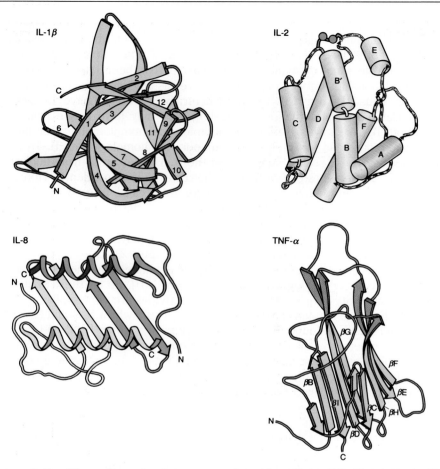

Figure 1.5. Three-dimensional structures of cytokines IL-1β (12), IL-2 (13), the IL-8 dimer (15), and single subunit of the TNFα trimer (14).

be more frequent on some cell lines. Density of expression and receptor affinity have been investigated using radiolabelled pure proteins. One of the earliest receptors to be elucidated was that of IL-2 (see Chapter 2). The fully functional high affinity receptor consists of two chains known as p75 and p55 both of which bind to IL-2. It is now apparent that, like IL-2, many other cytokine receptors, e.g. those for GM-CSF, IL-3, and IL-6, require co-operation between one or more protein chains to mediate high affinity cytokine binding (17).

The mechanism by which signals are transduced from receptor to nucleus are incompletely understood. There is evidence that calcium ions (Ca^{2+}), GTP and cyclic AMP, phospholipids, and protein kinases are involved. Via these mechanisms cytokines initiate the production of DNA binding proteins which bind to cytokine responsive elements leading to gene transcription.

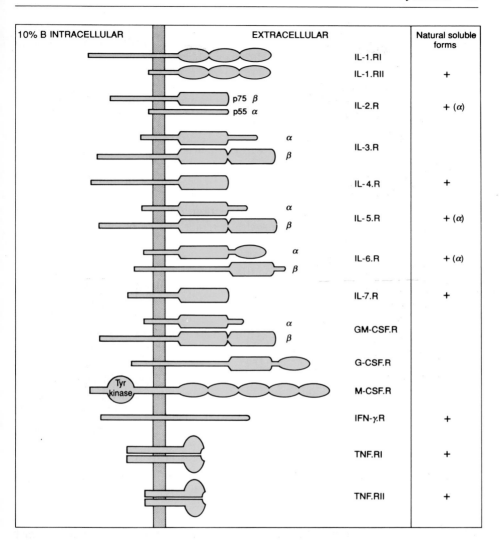

Figure 1.6. Cytokine receptors. The cytokine receptors display several structural motifs including immunoglobulin superfamily domains (◯) and a domain containing a WSXWS motif (▭). The TNF receptor is related to the NGF receptor, as well as the CD40 molecule. The WSXWS domain also occurs in receptors for prolactin, growth hormone and erythropoietin.

Not only do the cytokine receptors exist in a cell-bound form but some, e.g. TNF-R, IL-1R, IL-2R, IL-4R, IL-5R, IL-7R, and IFN-γR, are found in a soluble form in serum. These soluble forms arise either from proteolytic cleavage of the membrane receptor or from alternative splicing of receptor mRNA which produces a truncated version lacking the membrane spanning and cytoplasmic domains (16). Their natural function is thought to be that of inhibitors which limit cytokine activity *in vivo*. Soluble receptors (natural or synthesized) provide a way of regulating cytokine activity in diseases where they may contribute to the pathology (see Chapter 5).

General aspects of cytokine biology

From *in vitro* studies it is clear that cytokines are made by different cells (see *Table 1.3*) often in response to their activation. Some, like IL-2, seem to be made mainly by a restricted type of cell (i.e. T cells) whilst others, like IL-1 and IL-6, can be produced by very different cell types. Many cell lines produce cytokines *in vitro* constitutively or after activation. As far as the immune system goes, macrophages and T cells emerge as a major source of cytokines.

In vitro cloning of T cells in mice has shown that CD4$^+$ T helper (TH) cells may be divided into two subpopulations on the basis of the cytokines they make: the so-called TH1 cells make IL-2, LT, and IFN-γ and the so-called TH2 cells make IL-4, IL-5, IL-6, and IL-10. In addition, IFN-γ made by TH1 cells inhibits cytokine production by TH2 cells and IL-10 made by TH2 cells inhibits cytokine production by TH1 cells (18). The cytokine patterns and the interrelationship between these cells suggest they have mutually exclusive important biological activities (see Chapters 3 and 4) which may be important in immunopathology (see Chapter 5).

The target cells of cytokine action may also be restricted or of very diverse types (*Table 1.3*). Early cytokine research suggested that many cytokines might be pleiotropic, i.e. have multiple activities on different target cells (5), and the availability of recombinant cytokines has confirmed this. Thus, IL-1 acts on T cells and is considered important in the immune response to antigens, but also has inflammatory effects on a variety of target cells (19). It is a puzzle how one molecule can exert such very different effects on different target cells, but it may be that the same receptor uses different intracellular signalling pathways in different cells. Alternatively it may be that the cytokine-binding part of the receptor may associate with different comolecules on the surface leading to different signalling pathways (17). Such different signalling pathways might lead to different transcriptional events and thus biological outcome.

Other observed biological peculiarities of cytokines may also have their explanation at the cytokine receptor level. Thus cytokines which are structurally not very related, e.g. TNF and LT, exert very similar biological effects by binding to the same receptor. Presumably they share the structural motif which binds to the receptor but little else. Conversely, cytokines which are unrelated and which bind to distinct receptors, e.g. IL-1, IL-6, and TNF, sometimes share many similar biological activities (20). This may be because the distinct cytokine–receptor interactions use the same signalling mechanism within the cell.

An important aspect of cytokine activity is that they frequently work together, with each other or with another stimulant, to produce effects. Thus, for example,

Table 1.3   Principle cellular sources and targets of cytokines

Lymphokine	Cellular source	Cellular target
IFN-α	Leucocytes	Many cells
IFN-β	Fibroblasts and epithelial cells	Many cells
IFN-γ	T cells, natural killer (NK) cells	Macrophages, T cells, B cells, NK cells
IL-1α and β	Macrophages, endothelial cells, large granular lymphocytes. T and B cells, fibroblasts, epithelial cells, astrocytes, keratinocytes, osteoblasts	Thymocytes, neutrophils, hepatocytes, chondrocytes, muscle cells, endothelial cells, epidermal cells, osteocytes, macrophages, T cells, B cells, fibroblasts
IL-2	T cells _(TH1 T CD4+ cells)_	T cells, B cells, macrophages,
IL-3	T cells, mast cells	Multipotential stem cells, mast cells
IL-4	T cells, mast cells, bone marrow stromal cells _(TH2 T cells)_	T cells, mast cells, B cells, macrophages, haematopoietic progenitor cells
IL-5	T cells (mast cells, B cells)	Eosinophils, B cells (mouse)
IL-6	Fibroblasts, T cells, macrophages endothelial cells, keratinocytes, mast cells	B cells, thymocytes, hepatocytes, T cells
IL-7	Thymic stromal cells	Pro-B cells, pre-B cells, thymocytes, activated mature T cells
IL-8	Monocytes, endothelial cells, epithelial cells, fibroblasts, chondrocytes, hepatocytes keratinocytes, synoviocytes	Neutrophils, T cells, basophils
IL-9	T cells	CD4+ T cells, mast cells, erythroid progenitors (human)
IL-10	T cells (TH2 and TH0), macrophages, B cells	Macrophages, mast cells, NK cells
IL-11	Stromal cells	Haematopoietic progenitor cells
IL-12	T cells, B lymphoblastoid cells	T cells, NK cells, LAK cells
GM-CSF	T cells, endothelial cells, fibroblasts, macrophages, mast cells	Multipotential stem cells, mature neutrophils and monocyte/macrophages
M-CSF	Fibroblasts, monocytes, endothelial cells	Multipotential stem cells, monocyte/macrophages
G-CSF	Macrophages, fibroblasts, endothelial cells, mesothelial cells, T cells	Multipotential stem cells, granulocytes
TNF-α	Macrophages, T cells, thymocytes, B cells, NK cells	Tumour cells, transformed cell lines, fibroblasts, macrophages, osteoclasts, neutrophils, adipocytes, eosinophils, endothelial cells, chondrocytes, hepatocytes
LT	T cells	Tumour cells, transformed cell lines, neutrophils, osteoclasts
TGF-β	Platelets, activated macrophages, T cells, mesothelial cells, fetal hepatocytes, thymocytes	Endothelial cells, T cells, B cells, keratinocytes, hepatocytes, fibroblasts, haematopoietic progenitors, osteoblasts, smooth muscle cells

LT and IFN-γ have a potent synergistic effect in antiproliferative assays *in vitro* and antitumour effects *in vivo* (21) and IL-2 and IL-4 synergize to cause proliferation of T cell clones (22). It may be that the interaction of one cytokine with its receptor may prime a cell to become responsive to a second signal. Alternatively, the occupancy of two receptors may deliver the correct signal to allow the cell to respond. The activities of cytokines not only are often synergistic, but they may also be antagonistic. Thus TGF-β inhibits the production of IL-2 by T cell clones (23).

Much of our understanding of the biology of cytokines comes from investigation of their generation and assay *in vitro*. This obviously has the disadvantage of looking at complex interactions away from natural anatomical and physiological constraints. It is therefore possible that not all of the reported 'activities' may be seen *in vivo*. In real life the complex cytokine interactions, sometimes referred to as the cytokine network, will be influenced by other growth factors and physiological control mechanisms.

Cytokines have been frequently referred to as hormones in that they are produced by one cell and may act at a distant site. However, acting at a distant site is an unusual mode of action restricted to the body's response to inflammation and stress. More often cytokines act locally on neighbouring cells (paracrine action) or back on to the same cells (autocrine action). Their activity is more usually restricted to the tissue environment in which they are generated.

Detection of cytokines *in vitro* is either by immunoassay [radioimmunoassay (RIA), enzyme-linked immunosorbent assay (ELISA) or immunoradiometric assay (IRMA)] or by bioassay (24; *Table 1.4*; see also Clemens *et al.* and Balkwill in 'Further reading'). Immunoassays rely on the development of antibodies to each cytokine and are sensitive, reliable, quick, and easy. They have the disadvantage of detecting biologically inactive cytokines which are either denatured or broken into fragments, or which are bound to a specific inhibitor e.g. the IL-1 inhibitor (known as the IL-1 receptor antagonist protein or IRAP) or the soluble TNF receptor (see Chapter 2).

Bioassays are more laborious and often less specific because the cells used for the assay may respond to more than one cytokine. Thus, IL-4 has been found to cause stimulation of thymocytes or T cell clones (22) used in assays for IL-1 and IL-2, respectively, and TNF and LT are hardly distinguishable biologically (see Chapter 2). Furthermore, a cytokine may induce the production of other cytokines which may influence different cells in a mixed target cell population, or which may interfere positively or negatively with assays on homogeneous cells. Induction of one cytokine by another has often been described, e.g. IL-1 and TNF stimulate fibroblasts to produce IL-6 (25). However, the advantage of bioassays is that they do measure biological activity, at least within the assay being used. Specificity can be checked by the introduction of antibodies into the bioassay (26). A list of the common bioassays for cytokines is shown in *Table 1.4*, which is by no means exhaustive but exemplifies the range of assays which are used. In general, a combination of both immunoassay and bioassay provides the most valuable information on cytokine release under different conditions.

Table 1.4   Bioassays for cytokines[a]

IFN-α	Virus yield reduction
IFN-β	Inhibition of viral RNA and protein synthesis
IFN-γ	Cell growth inhibition
IL-1	Co-mitogenic stimulation of mouse thymocytes in presence of mitogen
	Proliferation of D10.64 T cell line
	Production of IL-2 by LBRM-33 or EL4.6.1 lines
	Production of fibroblast prostaglandin
	Bone resorbtion
	Proteoglycan release from cartilage
IL-2	Proliferation of IL-2-dependent T cell lines
IL-3	Haematopoietic colony formation from bone marrow
	Proliferation of IL-3-dependent lines
	Induction of 20α-steroid dehydrogenase in nude mouse spleen cells or bone marrow
IL-4	Co-stimulation of mouse splenic B cells in presence of anti-Ig
	Increase in Class II MHC expression by B cells
	Induction of IgG by T-depleted spleen cells
	Induction of IgE by T-depleted spleen cells
	Proliferation of cell lines (B e.g. BALM-4 or haematopoietic progenitors e.g. TF-1)
	Co-stimulation of T cells stimulated with PHA
IL-5	Induction of proliferation and IgM production by B cell lines (e.g. mouse[b] BCL-1 or human[b] TF-1)
	Proliferation or antibody secretion by large B cells (mouse)[b]
	Induction of secondary anti-DNP IgG antibody to DNP-primed T-depleted B cells (mouse)[b]
	Differentiation of eosinophil colonies in bone marrow or cord blood cultures
IL-6	Ig production by normal B cells (human)[b]
	Ig production by Epstein–Barr virus-transformed cell lines (human)[b]
	Proliferation of murine B9 cell line
IL-7	Proliferation of pre B cell-lines dependent on IL-7
IL-8	Chemokinesis or chemotaxis of polymorphonuclear leucocytes
IL-9	Growth of T cell lines
IL-10	Inhibition cytokine production by TH1 T cells
IL-11	Proliferation of IL-6-dependent cell line (T1165)
GM-CSF	
G-CSF	Haematopoietic colony formation of bone marrow cells
M-CSF	
TNF	
LT	Antiproliferative activity on certain tumour cell lines
TGF-β	Inhibition of proliferation of mink lung fibroblasts

[a] Reference 14 and Clemens *et al.* (1987) and Balkwill (1991) (Further reading).
[b] Indicates that assay only available for that species.

As an alternative to studying cytokine release it is possible to look for the availability of cytokine message within cells [see Balkwill (1991), in 'Further reading']. Whilst this indicates activation of the genes it does not provide information on translation of the message into protein and export from the cells to become biologically active. Nevertheless, Northern analysis and *in situ* hybridization have given useful information about cytokine gene activation in cells *in vitro* and *in vivo*.

Whilst the information gathered from *in vitro* work has provided enormous amounts of valuable information about the biological activity of cytokines it is obviously important to understand their biological functions *in vivo*. Several approaches are available. Injection of cytokines into animals or humans for therapeutic reasons has indicated the power and range of their biological activities (27). The creation of mice transgenic for cytokine genes has not only shown that the range of biological activities of some cytokines seen *in vitro* is reflected *in vivo*, but also in some circumstances has provided new insights (28). Thus mice made transgenic for the IL-6 gene had predictable alterations in immunoglobulin isotype switching and developed polyclonal plasmocytomas. However, they also had mesangial cell glomerulonephritis not previously predicted from *in vitro* work (29). The obverse of the transgenic animal in which genes are 'knocked out' or crippled is a further method to show the importance of a cytokine for biological function and indeed for the very existence of an animal. Recently mice have been described in which the IL-2, IL-4, IL-10, and LIF (leukaemia inhibitory factor) genes have been deleted (30). Whilst some of these animals, like the mice with IL-4 deleted, exhibited pathology predictable from *in vitro* and *in vivo* experimentation, others like the mice with LIF deleted showed unpredictable pathology (31,32). It remains to be seen what mechanisms surviving mice use to compensate for cytokine deletion and what response animals can make to infection.

Since cytokines are inducible, looking for cytokines in body fluids by bioassay and immunoassay and in tissues by *in situ* hybridization or immunocytochemical staining indicates cellular activation and provides insight into the nature of that activation. Similar techniques may be applied to analyse the expression of both cell-bound and soluble forms of cytokine receptors. Together these approaches are allowing analysis of the relevance of *in vitro* observations to circumstances *in vivo* and giving insights into the biology of cytokines.

Further reading

Balkwill, F. (ed.) (1991) *Cytokines—A practical approach*. IRL Press, Oxford.

Callard, R. E. and Gearing, A. J. H. (1994) *The cytokine facts book*. Academic Press, London.

Clemens, M. J., Morris, A. G., and Gearing, A. J. H. (eds) (1987) *Lymphokines and interferons—A practical approach*. IRL Press, Oxford

Foxwell, B. M. J., Barrett, K., and Feldman, M. (1992) Cytokine receptors; structure and signal transduction. *Clin. Exp. Immunol.*, **90**, 161.

Glover, D. M. (ed.) (1985–1987) *DNA cloning—A practical approach*. Vols. I–III, IRL Press, Oxford.

Meager, A. (1990) *Cytokines*. Open University Press, Milton Keynes.

Miyajima, A., Kitamura, T., Harada, N., Yokota, T., and Arai, K.-I. (1992) Cytokine receptors and signal transduction. *Annu. Rev. Immunol.*, **10**, 295.

Oppenheim, J. J. and Shevach, E. M. (eds) (1991) *Immunophysiology; the role of cells and cytokines in immunity and inflammation*. Oxford University Press, Oxford.

Thomson, A., (ed.) (1991) *The cytokine handbook*. Academic Press, London.

References

1. Bennett,B. and Bloom,B.R. (1968) *Proc. Natl. Acad. Sci. USA*, **59**, 756.
2. Kasakura,S. and Lowenstein,L. (1970) *J. Immunol.*, **105**, 1162.
3. Bloom,B.R. and Bennett,B. (1966) *Science*, **153**, 180.
4. Dumonde,D.C., Wolstencroft,R.A., Panayi,G.S., Mathew,M., Morley,J., and Howson,W.T. (1969) *Nature*, **224**, 38.
5. Waksman,B.H. (1979) In *Biology of the lymphokines* (ed. S.Cohen, E.Pick, and J.J.Oppenheim). Academic Press, New York, p. 585.
6. Cohen,S. *et al.* (1977) *Cell. Immunol.*, **33**, 233.
7. Aarden,L.A. *et al.* (1979) *J. Immunol.*, **123**, 2928.
8. Paul,W.E., Kishimoto,T., Melchers,F., Metcalf,D., Mosmann,T., Oppenheim,J., Ruddle,N., and Van Snick,J. (1992) *Clin. Exp. Immunol.*, **88**, 367.
9. Yoshida,T. (1979) In *Biology of the lymphokines* (ed. S.Cohen, E.Pick, and J.J.Oppenheim). Academic Press, New York, p. 259.
10. Contreras,R. Demolder, J., and Fiers,W. (1991) In *Cytokines—A practical approach* (ed. F.R.Balkwill). IRL Press, Oxford, p. 1.
11. Sanderson,C.J., Campbell,H.D., and Young,I.G. (1988) *Immunol. Rev.*, **102**, 29.
12. Priestle,J.P., Shär,H.-P., and Grütter,M.G. (1988) *EMBO J.*, **7**, 339.
13. Brandhuber,B.J., Boone,T., Kenney,W.C., and McKay,D.B. (1987) *Science*, **238**, 1707.
14. Jones,E.Y., Stuart,D.I., and Walker,N.P.C. (1989) *Nature*, **338**, 225.
15. Clore,G.M., Appella,E., Yamada,M., Matsushima,K., and Gronenborn,A.M. (1990) *Biochemistry*, **29**, 1689.
16. Gillis,S. (1991) *Curr. Opin. Immunol.*, **3**, 315.
17. Nicola,N.A. and Metcalf,D. (1991) *Cell*, **67**, 1.
18. Mosmann,T.R. and Coffman,R.L. (1989) *Annu. Rev. Immunol.*, **7**, 145.
19. Oppenheim,J.J., Kovacs,E.J., Matsushima,K., and Duram,S.K. (1986) *Immunol. Today*, **7**, 45.
20. Dinarello,C.A. (1991) *Blood*, **77**, 1627.
21. Stone-Wolff,D.S., Yip,Y.K., Kelker,H.C., Lee,J., Henriksen-De Stefano,D., Rubin,B.Y., Rinderknecht,E., Aggarwal,B.B., and Vilcek,J. (1984) *J. Exp. Med.*, **159**, 828.
22. Spits,H., Yssel,H., Takebe,Y., Arai,N., Yokota,T., Lee,F., Arai,K., Banchereau,J., and de Vries,J.E. (1987) *J. Immunol.*, **139**, 1142.
23. Lucas,C., Wallick,S., Fendly,B.M., Figari,I., and Palladino,A. (1991) In *Clinical applications of TGF-β*. (ed. G.R.Bock and J.Marsh). Ciba Foundation Symposium, vol. **157**, p. 98, John Wiley and Sons, Chichester.
24. Hamblin,A.S. and O'Garra,A. (1987) In *Lymphocytes—A practical approach* (ed. G.G.B.Klaus). IRL Press, Oxford, p. 209.
25. Van-Damme,J., Opdenakker,G., Simpson,R.J., Rubira,M.R., Cayphas,S., Vink,A., Billiau,A., and Van Snick,J. (1987) *J. Exp. Med.*, **165**, 914.
26. Cherwinski,H.M., Schumacher,J.H., Brown,K.D., and Mosmann,T.R. (1987) *J. Exp. Med.*, **166**, 1229.
27. Balkwill,F.R. (1989) *Cytokines in cancer therapy*. Oxford University Press, Oxford.
28. Hanahan,D. (1989) *Science*, **246**, 1265.
29. Suematsu,S., Matsuda,T., Aozasa,K., Akira,S., Nakano,N., Ohno,S., Miyazaki,J., Yamamura,K., Hirano,T., and Kishimoto,T. (1989) *Proc. Natl. Acad. Sci. USA*, **30**, 7547.
30. Paul,W.E. (1992) *Nature*, **357**, 16.
31. Stewart,C.L., Kaspar,P., Brunet,L.J., Bhatt,H., Gadi,I., Köntgen,F., and Abbondanzo,S.J. (1992) *Nature*, **359**, 76.
32. Heath,J.K. (1992) *Nature*, **359**, 17.

2

Cytokines one by one

The interferons

Interferons are inducible proteins which are important not only in defence against a wide range of viruses but also in the regulation of immune responses in haematopoietic cell development (*Table 2.1*). Whilst there is only one IFN-γ and one IFN-β gene there are at least 23 different genetic loci for the α interferons of which 15 correspond to functional genes. IFN-α_1 genes encode proteins of 165–166 amino acids while IFN-α_2 genes encode glycosylated proteins of 172 amino acids (1); all IFN-α subtypes are synthesized in humans with a 23 amino acid signal sequence which is cleaved off. Human IFN-β contains 166 amino acids preceded by a 21 amino acid signal sequence and is only 30% homologous with IFN-α at the amino acid level and 45% at the nucleotide level. Unusually for cytokines both IFN-α and -β genes lack introns. Unlike IFN-α, IFN-β has one *N*-glycosylated site. IFN-α and -β share a common receptor the distribution of which is ubiquitous. The gene for this receptor is located on chromosome 21 (2).

IFN-α and -β are produced by most cells in response to viral infection or

Table 2.1 Biological activities of interferons

	IFN-α	IFN-β	IFN-γ
Enhances or inhibits cell differentiation	+	−	+
Enhances Class I MHC expression	+	+	+
Induces or enhances Class II MHC expression	−	−	+
Activates macrophages	−	−	+
Enhances NK cell activity	+	+	+
Enhances B cell proliferation and maturation	−	−	+
Increases secretion of other cytokines	−	−	+
Increases cell surface receptors for Fcγ and cytokines	−	−	+
Inhibits normal and transformed cell growth	+	+	+
Protects cells from viruses	+	+	+
Counteracts effects of IL-4 on B cells	−	−	+

stimulation with natural or synthetic double-stranded RNA such as poly(I:C). They have potent antiviral activity but at higher concentration have antiproliferative activity against both normal and tumour cells. They can enhance the expression of Class I MHC gene products and enhance natural killer (NK) cell activity and thus play a role in immunoregulation. These activities have been exploited therapeutically for the treatment of viral infections and tumours.

IFN-γ has potent immunoregulatory effects on a variety of cells (*Table 2.1*) including activation of macrophages, induction of FcγRI on macrophages and FcγRII on granulocytes, enhanced production of IgG2a by B lymphocytes, and enhanced expression of Class I MHC gene products and Class II MHC gene products. It can also induce *de novo* expression of Class II MHC gene products on most cells *in vitro*, thus rendering them able to participate in Class II mediated immune reactions. IFN-γ counteracts the effects of IL-4 on B cells and thus inhibits the activity of TH2 cells (3). It is produced by T lymphocytes from blood or lymphoid tissues upon stimulation with specific antigens, mitogens, or allo-antigens. Both CD4$^+$ and CD8$^+$ T lymphocytes and NK cells can produce IFN-γ, although the TH1 CD4$^+$ cells are considered the major producers in response to antigens (3).

Size fractionation of human IFN-γ produced by mitogen stimulation of peripheral blood leucocytes was by molecular sieving and suggested two forms with pIs (using isoelectric focusing) of 8.3 and 8.5 and molecular weights of 20 and 25 kDa. These two forms are the products of a single gene on chromosome 12 in the human (4) and 10 in the mouse (5) with size and charge differences arising from differences in glycosylation at residue 25 (both forms) and 97 (25 kDa form) of the polypeptide sequence. IFN-γ secreted by activated T cells is mostly in the form of a homodimer of the 25 kDa subunits. The extent of glycosylation is variable but biological activity is unaffected by this; recombinant IFN-γ prepared in *Escherichia coli* is biologically active. The human cDNA codes for 166 amino acids of which the first 23 have the characteristics of a signal sequence (6). The secreted protein consists of 143 amino acids and has a structure unrelated to that of IFN-α or -β suggesting that it has independent evolutionary origins. Amongst the various other species examined, there is little sequence homology at the amino acid level, which probably explains the lack of cross-species activity.

A specific receptor for human IFN-γ has been characterized which is distinct from the receptor for IFN-α and -β. The gene has been cloned and is located on the long arm of chromosome 6 (7,8) and contains a number of cysteine residues (*Figure 1.6*) with a molecular size of 117 kDa. The receptor is widely distributed on different cell types and to date all human cells tested have been shown to bear receptors. There are about 100–10 000 receptors per cell which bind IFN-γ with high affinity (K$_d$ of $3–10 \times 10^{-9}$ M). Experiments suggest another cell surface protein is needed for adequate signal transduction by the receptor. Binding of IFN-γ to its receptor leads to rapid internalization of the complex at 37°C by receptor-mediated endocytosis. The induction of several proteins associated with the antiviral state and immunoregulation follows induction of a second message which acts on the interferon-responsive sequences in the non-coding portion of the genes leading to their transcription (9). Increased *de novo* synthesis of between 50 and 100 proteins by the stimulated cell occurs alongside inhibition of others. The changes in the cells exposed to IFN-γ alters their reactivity within the immune system.

Interleukin 1

Interleukin 1 (IL-1) is a polypeptide with diverse roles in immunity and inflammation (see Chapters 3 and 4) having both protective and proinflammatory effects (10). A list of the diverse biological activities of IL-1 are shown in *Table 2.2*.

Table 2.2   Biological activities of IL-1

Cofactor for T cell activation
Cofactor for B cell activation
Promotes haematopoiesis
Mediates fever
Promotes breakdown of cartilage and bone
Activates neutrophils
Activates vascular endothelial cells
Induces acute phase protein release
Induces proteolysis of muscle cells
Induces cytokine synthesis
Mitogenic for fibroblasts

IL-1 is synthesized by many cell types but particularly monocytes and macrophages which have been activated. These cells are potent producers of IL-1 upon stimulation with a variety of agents including endotoxin, muramyl dipeptide, phorbol myristate acetate (PMA), and silica. Unstimulated monocytes possess low levels of mRNA for IL-1 which rise 2 h after stimulation, followed at 3 h by IL-1 protein which is detectable outside the cell.

Early work suggested that many of the bioactivities in *Table 1.1* co-purified with a molecule of molecular weight 16–17 kDa (11). Further characterization of natural IL-1 demonstrated biologically active molecules of higher and lower molecular weight in culture supernatants and body fluids which showed charge heterogeneity with a major species having a pI of 7 and a minor species having a pI of 5 (12). Cloning of the genes for IL-1 revealed that there are two related gene products corresponding to these pIs, known as IL-1α and IL-1β (13). Most human IL-1 secreted by stimulated macrophages is IL-1β, corresponding to the species of pI 7.0 whilst IL-1α corresponds to the minor secreted IL-1 species at pI 5.

The IL-1s do not contain the hydrophobic signal sequences which are normally associated with the transport of molecules across membranes. IL-1s are synthesized as large precursor molecules (31 kDa) which are cleaved by serine proteases to give the 17.5 kDa mature proteins. Whilst several common enzymes can cleave the precursors, one protease seems to be specific for IL-1β and is known as the IL-1β converting enzyme (ICE). The majority of IL-1α precursors remains in the cytosol. Some IL-1α may be membrane-associated where it is biologically active (14). Biologically active fragments of IL-1 which have been recovered from body fluids such as plasma and urine may represent further breakdown products of the mature protein (14).

The genes for IL-1α and IL-1β are similarly organized. The genes code for precursor proteins of 271 (IL-1α) and 269 (IL-1β) amino acids. Human IL-1β is 27% homologous with IL-1α at the amino acid level, the homology occurring mainly at the carboxyl-terminus. Thus IL-1α and -β are the products of two independently evolving genes with differing but related protein structures and similar biological activities. A crystallographic study of IL-1β suggests that the structure is probably tetrahedral and composed of 12 β-bands complexed by hydrogen bonds (*Figure 1.5*).

There are two IL-1 receptors (IL-1RI and IL-1RII) both of which are members of the immunoglobulin supergene family (10,14; *Figure 1.6*). IL-1RI is found on T and B cells, fibroblasts, keratinocytes, endothelial cells, chondrocytes, hepato-cytes, and synovial lining cells and has a molecular weight of 80 kDa. IL-1RII is found on B cells, neutrophils, and bone-marrow cells and has a molecular weight of 60 kDa. The difference in molecular weight arises from IL-1RII having a shorter cytosolic region. There is some evidence that these two receptors can mediate different biological events even though they both bind the two IL-1s (10, 14).

A number of proteins inhibit the activity of IL-1. These include lipoproteins, lipid, and α-2 macroglobulin although the effects are not specific for IL-1. There is, however, a polypeptide which inhibits IL-1 specifically known as the IL-1 receptor antagonist protein (IRAP), a 23–25 kDa protein originally purified from the urine of patients with monocytic leukaemia and subsequently cloned, which has 26% amino acid homology to IL-1β and 19% homology to IL-1α. It competes with the binding of both IL-1s to their cell surface receptors, and has been shown to block the activity of IL-1 in various models of disease in animals and *in vitro* (10,14).

Interleukin 2

T cell growth factor (TCGF), now known as IL-2, is a polypeptide produced by activated T cells which acts on T cells to promote their division and activation of other cells of the immune system such as NK and B cells (15; *Table 2.3*). Human IL-2 was first purified from the culture supernatants of mitogen- or alloantigen-activated T cells and the leukaemic cell line Jurkat, and was shown to have a molecular weight of 14–17 kDa on SDS–PAGE.

The cDNA consists of a single open reading frame coding for 153 amino acids (*Figure 1.4*). The first 20 amino acids of the amino-terminal end are hydrophobic and constitute the signal sequence which is cleaved off to give the mature protein

Table 2.3 Biological activities of IL-2

Stimulates T cell proliferation
Stimulates B cell growth and differentiation
Generates lymphokine-activated killer (LAK) cells
Activates macrophages
Stimulates T cells to produce other cytokines
Stimulates proliferation of oligodendrocytes

which consists of 133 amino acids and a predicted molecular weight of 15 kDa. The natural product is *O*-glycosylated at the threonine residue at position 3 of the mature molecule.

There is a single copy of the human gene consisting of four exons and three introns on chromosome 4 in the human (16) (*Figure 2.1*). The IL-2 molecule contains a single disulphide bond between residues 58 and 105 and chemical

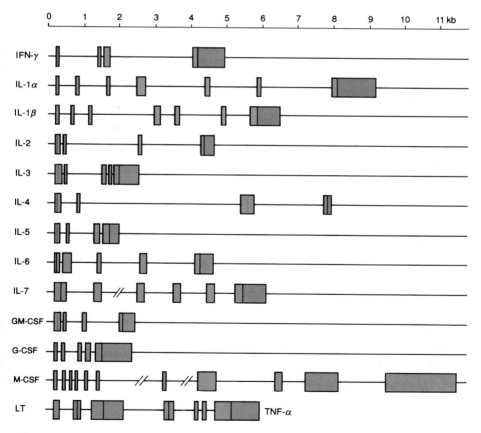

Figure 2.1.   Genomic organization of cytokine genes showing exons (solid orange) and introns (single lines). The 3′ and 5′ untranslated regions are shown in grey.

reduction of the bond or site-directed mutagenesis of these residues leads to loss of biological activity showing that the bond is essential for bioactivity. The complete tertiary structure of IL-2 has been determined from X-ray crystallography and consists of six α-helical regions (*Figure 1.5*).

IL-2 interacts with cells by binding to a receptor of which there are two forms with differing affinities; a high affinity receptor (K_d 1×10^{-11} M) which mediates the physiological response of T cells to IL-2 and a low affinity receptor (K_d 1×10^{-8} M) which does not. Determination of the number of receptor sites per cell by binding studies with either radio-iodinated IL-2 or an anti-receptor antibody (known as anti-Tac) produced discrepant results, the latter giving higher values than the former (17). The explanation for this became clear once the gene for a 55 kDa receptor protein (α chain) was cloned and transfected into other cells. Transfection of non-lymphoid cells with this human IL-2 receptor gene produced low affinity receptors whereas transfection of T cell lines produced high and low affinity receptors (18). This raised the possibility that lymphocytes coded for a second IL-2 binding protein which could interact with the 55 kDa molecule to give rise to high affinity receptors. A second molecule with a molecular weight of 75 kDa (β chain) has been cloned which binds IL-2 with an affinity intermediate between that of low and high affinity (19) and is a member of the haematopoietin receptor family (*Figure 1.6*). A third chain with a molecular weight 64 kDa has recently been cloned (IL-2Rγ) and has been shown to have protein kinase activity and to be concerned with signal transduction (20). The high affinity receptors are therefore composed of at least two subunits, each of which can independently bind IL-2 with lower affinity. Each subunit of the receptor may interact with a different region of the IL-2 molecule and the binding of IL-2 to both proteins produces the biologically active high affinity receptor (21) (*Figure 2.2*).

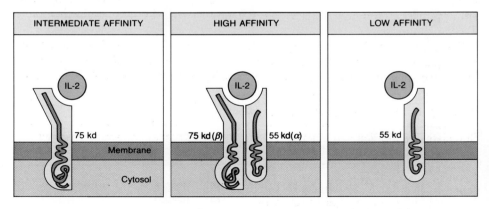

Figure 2.2.   IL-2 receptors. The high affinity IL-2 receptor is formed from two non-covalently linked polypeptides, each of which has some affinity for IL-2. The larger (75 kDa) peptide contains a longer intracytoplasmic section which is thought to be involved in signalling, while the smaller (55 kDa) peptide is recognized by the anti-TAC monoclonal antibody and is now referred to as CD25.

IL-2 production and high affinity receptor expression are transient events associated with T cell activation (22) (see Chapter 3). The 75 kDa molecule is expressed on resting T cells as well as NK cells (23). However, the 55 kDa molecule is induced on activation and when expressed on the cell surface with the 75 kDa molecule gives rise to the high affinity receptor. Binding of IL-2 to the 75 kDa molecule is able to initiate induction of the gene transcribing the 55 kDa molecule and hence development of a functional high affinity receptor. However, cells such as NK cells, which have been reported to be CD25 (IL-2Rα) negative, but which proliferate in response to IL-2, may do so by stimulation through the 75 kDa molecule alone (21,23). The intracellular region of the 75 kDa molecule consisting of 286 amino acids has a triplet of amino acids implicated as the catalytic domain of some protein kinases.

Interleukin 3

Interleukin 3 (IL-3) is a haematopoietic growth factor which supports the growth and differentiation of pluripotent stem cells leading to different blood cell types, particularly erythroid and myeloid cells (24; *Table 2.4*). IL-3 is produced by activated T helper lymphocytes and by mast cells and is constitutively produced by some cell lines like the murine WEH1-3B cell line. The constitutive production of IL-3 by this line is associated with the insertion of a retrovirus close to the 5′ end of the IL-3 gene (see Chapter 5). Whilst IL-3 stimulates the production of myeloid cell progenitors *in vitro* it is unclear how it might affect their growth *in vivo* since it is produced principally by T cells and not by the cells in the stroma of the bone marrow. It is undetectable in serum except when there is massive T cell stimulation as there is in graft versus host disease. From these findings it is believed that IL-3 is a link between the immune and haematopoietic system, stimulating recruitment of cells from the bone-marrow when there is activation of T cells and mast cells.

The cDNA clones encoding murine IL-3 were described in 1984 (25) whilst the corresponding human sequence remained unknown until 1986, when a cDNA clone encoding IL-3 was isolated from a gibbon T cell line (26). This gibbon

Table 2.4   Biological activities of IL-3

Stimulates generation and differentiation of progenitor cells of various lineages from pluripotent stem cells (i.e. monocyte, granulocyte, basophils, eosinophils mast cells, erythroid cells, and megakaryocytes) *in vitro*
Stimulates haematopoiesis *in vivo*
Induces Thy-1 expression on lymphocytes
Prolongs survival of mucosal mast cells
Induces limited division and enhances phagocytosis of macrophages
Activates basophils
Stimulates antibody-dependent cellular cytotoxicity (ADCC) phagocytosis, and superoxide production by eosinophils

cDNA was used as a hybridization probe for the human gene. The human gene for IL-3 is located on chromosome 5 (*Figure 2.1*) and encodes a protein of 152 amino acids of which 19 amino acids are the signal sequence (26). It has two potential glycosylation sites and two cysteine residues involved in one disulphide bond between residues 16 and 84. The exon/intron arrangement is similar to that in the mouse gene but there is only 29% homology between the human and mouse proteins.

The IL-3 receptor consists of at least two subunits which are members of the haematopoietin supergene family of receptors, an α chain which binds IL-3 specifically, and a β chain which confers high affinity (27; *Figure 1.6*).

Interleukin 4

Interleukin 4 (IL-4) causes activation, proliferation, and differentiation of B cells, is also a growth factor for T cells and mast cells, and exerts other effects on granulocyte, megakaryocyte, and erythrocyte precursors and macrophages (28–31; *Table 2.5*). IL-4 regulates B cell growth and expression of cell surface antigens such as CD23 and Class II MHC which it upregulates. It is a switch factor for IgE and IgG1 by B lymphocytes (see Chapter 3). The major source of IL-4 is the activated TH2 subset of CD4$^+$ T cells in mice (3) and the equivalent population in humans.

Table 2.5   Biological activities of IL-4

On B lymphocytes
Induces proliferation in the presence of anti-IgM or SAC (*Staphylococcus aureus* Cowan strain 1)
Induces MHC Class II expression
Increases cell volume
Induces expression and release of low affinity IgE receptor (CD23)
Stimulates IgG1 and IgE synthesis
Inhibits IgM, IgG3, IgG2a, and IgG2b synthesis

On T lymphocytes
Induces proliferation of thymocytes
Enhances proliferation of PHA-activated mature lymphocytes
Enhances cytotoxic activity of CTLs
Inhibits IL-2-induced CTL and LAK activity

On other cells
Stimulates mast cell growth
Activates haemopoietic progenitor cell growth
Induces macrophage aggregation, migration inhibition, and cytotoxicity
Induces MHC Class I and II expression and tumouricidal activity of macrophages
Inhibits stromal cell support for haematopoietic colony formation
Downregulates the expression of CD23 on macrophages
Blocks IL-1, IL-6, IL-8, and TNF-α production and stimulates G-CSF and M-CSF production by monocytes

A clone was isolated from a human cDNA library prepared from a concanavalin-A-stimulated T cell line (31). This codes for a protein of 153 amino acids of which the first 24 constitute a signal sequence. Human IL-4 is inactive on mouse cells as is mouse IL-4 on human. The human IL-4 gene (*Figure 2.1*) is located on chromosome 5 with other cytokine genes for IL-3, IL-5, GM-CSF, M-CSF, and the M-CSFR.

Receptors for IL-4 are found on virtually every cell tested so far including T and B cells, monocytes, fibroblasts, myeloid epithelial and endothelial cells. The protein binds IL-4 with a single high affinity and has a molecular weight of around 130 kDa. There are approximately 300 receptors on B and T cells but more on B cell lymphomas and T cell lines. Receptor numbers increase on cell activation. The human IL-4 receptor is a member of the haematopoietin receptor family (*Figure 1.6*) (27,29,32). Alternative splicing leads to a receptor without the transmembrane or cytosolic portions which is a soluble form of the receptor and which may be a natural inhibitor of IL-4 activity.

Interleukin 5

Interleukin 5 (IL-5) causes B-cell activation, growth, and differentiation (see Chapter 3) as well as eosinophil differentiation (33,34). It is this latter activity which in humans seems to be particularly important. Proliferation and terminal differentiation of eosinophil precursors is dependent on IL-5. It also increases the survival time of eosinophils in parasitic infection and activates mature eosinophils (*Table 2.6*).

Natural murine IL-5 purified as a protein of molecular weight 42–66 kDa, which is reduced to 40 kDa on SDS–PAGE. The murine cDNA codes for 133 amino acids with a signal sequence of 18 amino acids (35). The human cDNA codes for a 134 amino acid protein of which the first 22 are the predicted signal sequence (36). There is 67% homology at the amino acid level between mouse and human IL-5. It is important to note that whilst murine recombinant IL-5 causes both B cell growth and eosinophil differentiation, the human recombinant homologue only causes eosinophil differentiation (34; see Chapter 4).

The specific IL-5 receptor (α chain) is a member of the haematopoietin receptor gene family (*Figure 1.6*). This chain, which binds IL-5 specifically but

Table 2.6   Biological activities of IL-5

Enhances proliferation of preactivated B cells[a]
Induces B cell differentiation[a]
Enhances IgA production[a]
Promotes eosinophil growth and differentiation
Activates mature eosinophils
Increases eosinophil survival in parasitic infections

[a] Mouse only; not in humans.

with low affinity, associates with another transmembrane protein, also a member of the haematopoietin receptor gene family. It is used as part of other cytokine receptors, such as those for GM-CSF and IL-3. The two chains bind IL-5 with high affinity (27,37,38).

Interleukin 6

Interleukin 6 (IL-6) is a terminal differentiation factor for B cells, a hybridoma/plasmacytoma growth factor and pro-inflammatory factor (39; *Table 2.7*). IL-6 shares several activities with IL-1 and TNF. It is synthesized by an enormous variety of cells (*Table 1.3*). Purified from natural sources it behaves as a single chain of molecular mass 21–28 kDa (40). The human cDNA predicts a protein of 212 amino acids including a 28 residue signal sequence (41).

Table 2.7   Biological activities of IL-6

Co-stimulates T cells and thymocytes
Induces B cell differentiation
Promotes growth of hybridomas
Stimulates acute-phase protein production by hepatocytes
Protects cells from viral infection (weakly)
Autocrine growth factor for myelomas
Competence factor to confer responsiveness to
    haematopoietic growth factors
Induces differentiation of CTLs
Induces fever (rabbits)

The IL-6 receptor is found on both lymphoid and non-lymphoid cells although expression may depend on the state of differentiation or activation of the cells e.g. normal resting B cells do not express IL-6Rs whilst activated B blasts do. Like the IL-2, IL-3 and IL-5 receptors, the IL-6 receptor consists of at least two chains, an α chain of molecular weight 80 kDa and a β chain of 130 kDa (24). The α chain has features of the haematopoietin family with an amino-terminal loop characteristic of the immunoglobulin supergene family (42; *Figure 1.6*). The intracellular domain is small. In contrast, the β chain, which is a member of the haematopoietin receptor family, has a longer intracellular domain involved in signalling. The β chain does not bind IL-6 unless the α chain is present and is also used as part of the IL-11 receptor (43).

Interleukin 7

Interleukin 7 (IL-7) is a growth factor for both B and T progenitors (44,45) and is thus important in lymphopoiesis. It is produced by stromal cells of the bone marrow and thymus. It also co-stimulates mature T cells (*Table 2.8*). The human

Table 2.8   Biological activities of IL-7

Promotes growth of pro-B cells
Promotes growth of thymocytes
Co-stimulates mature T cells

cDNA encodes molecule of 177 amino acids of which 25 form the signal sequence (46). Human IL-7 is highly homologous to mouse IL-7 (60%).

Isolation of both human and mouse IL-7 receptor cDNAs have been reported; in addition to the membrane form of the receptor, a secreted form has been described (47). The IL-7 receptor is a member of the haematopoietin receptor gene family (27; *Figure 1.6*).

Interleukin 8 and the chemokines

It is now apparent that there is a group of cytokines which are related in terms of both sequence and genomic structure. These have been called by different workers the 'small cytokine' or scy family (48), intercrines (49) or chemokines, the last now being their agreed title. A list of these proteins is shown in *Table 2.9*. All are around 8–10 kDa in size. The proteins may be separated into two distinctive subgroups based on whether the first two of the four position-invariant cysteine residues common among the various primary sequences are adjacent (C-C or β subgroup) or separated by another amino acid (C-X-C or α subgroup). Structural analysis has shown that the cysteine residues are important for the tertiary structure of the proteins. Amino acid analysis shows the proteins contain leader sequences suggesting they are secreted by conventional pathways. In the human genes for the C-C subgroup are located on chromosome 17 and those for the C-X-C subgroup on chromosome 4.

The IL-8 gene encodes a 99 amino acid precursor molecule which contains a 20 amino acid signal sequence. The secreted protein is processed by proteases to give several biologically active forms of which that containing 72 amino acids is

Table 2.9   Chemokine superfamily members

C-X-C subgroup (α family)

Interleukin 8 (IL-8)
Melanoma growth stimulatory activity (MGSA; GRO α,β and γ)
Platelet factor 4 (PF4)
β-thromboglobulin (βTG)

C-C subgroup (β family)

Macrophage chemotactic and activating factor (MCAF)
RANTES
LD-8/MIP-1α
ACT-2/MIP-1β

the major one. The three-dimensional structure has been elucidated (50) and the molecule seems to occur as a dimer with a structure closely related to folding of the α1 and α2 domains of the MHC Class I antigen HLA-A2 (*Figure 1.5*).

IL-8 receptors on neutrophils seem to be of a single type with high affinity binding and there are around 20 000 per neutrophil. The receptor has been cloned (51,52) and has been shown to be a member of the rhodopsin superfamily of receptors, which have seven transmembrane hydrophobic regions that are coupled to guanine nucleotide binding proteins (G proteins). All C-X-C related cytokines compete for IL-8 binding to its receptor and MCAF and MIP-1α can compete for RANTES binding. Such interactions may be important in the development of cytokine cascades.

IL-8 is made by both leucocytes and non-leucocytes (*Table 1.3*). Originally described as a chemoattractant for neutrophils but not for monocytes, it has also now been shown to activate them causing degranulation, increase in respiratory burst, mobilization of intracellular Ca^{2+} stores, increased lysosomal enzyme release, increased adherence to unstimulated endothelial monolayers, and increased expression of CR1 and CD11/CD18. IL-8 is also chemotactic for T cells and basophils although less effectively than for neutrophils. *In vivo* this cytokine causes a neutrophilia when administered intravenously and plasma exudation and neutrophil infiltration into tissues which is maintained for some hours when administered locally (*Table 2.10*).

Table 2.10   Biological activities of IL-8

Chemoattractive for neutrophils, T cells, and basophils
Activates neutrophils
Stimulates adhesion of monocytes to endothelial cells
Stimulates proliferation of keratinocytes
Induces neutrophilia *in vivo*

The other chemokines also have multiple activities on multiple targets and are produced by a variety of cells. They have functions which are important in inflammatory modulation of haematopoiesis, tissue repair, and regulation of immune function. The C-X-C family contains other chemotactic cytokines (GRO-α, -β, and -γ) as does the C-C family (RANTES, MIP-1α, and 1β). The final number of members of this family and their physiological function has yet to be fully determined.

Interleukin 9

Interleukin 9 (IL-9), also known as T cell growth factor p40 in the mouse, was originally isolated on the basis of its ability to support the growth of certain mouse helper T cell clones. It was also shown to enhance mast cell activity and mast cell growth in the presence of IL-3 and IL-4 (53). The human homologue

Table 2.11   Biological activities of IL-9

Stimulates T cell proliferation
Enhances mast cell growth and activity
Stimulates erythroid colony formation

has these activities but also stimulates erythroid colony formation *in vitro* suggesting it may play a role in normal haematopoiesis (*Table 2.11*). The human gene is found on the long arm of chromosome 5 near the genes for IL-3, IL-4, IL-5, and GM-CSF with which it shares regulatory elements. The cDNA encodes an 144 amino acid protein of 16 kDa containing an 18 amino acid signal sequence. The protein has four glycosylation sites and 10 cysteine residues which are conserved in mouse and man (55). The receptor for IL-9 is a 64 kDa member of the haematopoietin receptor superfamily.

Many of the *in vitro* actions of IL-9 overlap with IL-3 and GM-CSF. It is produced particularly by CD4 T cells and stimulates their growth. In this respect it differs from IL-2 and IL-4 in supporting T cell growth in the absence of APCs.

Interleukin 10

This cytokine, formerly known as cytokine synthesis inhibitory factor, is a product of TH2 T cells, as well as monocytes, macrophages, and B cells, which inhibits cytokine production and proliferation by mouse TH1 and TH0 T cells (3). It does this by acting on antigen-presenting macrophages but not B cells or dendritic cells (56), causing them to downregulate Class II MHC expression. IL-10 also enhances the proliferative responses of T cells to IL-2 and IL-4, is a cytotoxic T cell differentiation factor, has mast cell growth stimulatory activity, and inhibits interferon production by NK cells (57) as well as having many other effects on various cells (*Table 2.12*).

The human cDNA encodes a 178 amino acid protein which has an 18 amino acid signal sequence, and has one potential *N*-glycosylation sites and four cysteine residues. Human and mouse IL-10 are 73% homologous at the amino acid level. The secreted protein exists as an acid-sensitive homodimer of 35–40 kDa.

Table 2.12   Biological activities of IL-10

Inhibits cytokine production by TH1 cells
Enhances T cell proliferation in the presence of IL-2 and IL-4
Enhances differentiation of cytotoxic T cells
Stimulates mast cell growth
Inhibits IFN production by NK cells
Inhibits Class II MHC and adhesion molecule expression and
    cytokine production by monocytes and macrophages
Enhances Class II MHC expression on B cells
Enhances proliferation and differentiation of activated B cells

The cDNA shows extensive homology with an open reading frame from Epstein–Barr virus and has led to the hypothesis that the virus may have captured the IL-10 gene and that this may give a selective advantage for the virus by suppressing the host's immune response.

Interleukin 11

Interleukin 11 (IL-11) is a cytokine which regulates the growth kinetics of various haematopoietic progenitor cells. It acts synergistically with other cytokines (IL-3, IL-4, and *steel* factor) to support the proliferation of early progenitors (58; *Table 2.13*). It has many properties similar to IL-6 such as the ability to stimulate the proliferation of plasmacytomas, T cell-dependent antibody formation by B cells, and human and murine megakaryocyte formation. IL-11 was initially identified in the culture supernatants from a primate bone marrow stromal cell line and subsequently from a human fetal lung fibroblast line (59,60). Human and primate IL-11 are 97% homologous at the nucleotide level.

Table 2.13   Biological properties of IL-11

Stimulates proliferation of plasmacytoma cells
Stimulates T-dependent development of antibody production
    by B cells
Stimulates megakaryocyte colony formation
Synergizes with IL-3 and IL-4 to support the proliferation of
    early bone-marrow progenitors

Interleukin 12

Interleukin 12 (IL-12) exerts a number of effects on T and NK cells (61–62; *Table 2.14*). It is a heterodimer consisting of two disulphide-bonded subunits of 40 and 35 kDa each encoded by different genes (63). Site-directed mutagenesis has shown that the disulphide bonds are essential for biological activity. The 35 kDa protein is homologous to IL-6 and G-CSF. These structural findings have led to speculation that IL-12 is a complex of cytokine and a soluble receptor which bind to gp130 or a gp130-like molecule on the surface of IL-12 responsive cells (64).

Table 2.14   Biological properties of IL-12

Augments antigen-specific cytotoxic T cell responses
Acts as a growth factor for T cells and NK cells.
Induces IFN and TNF secretion by T cells and NK cells
Enhances expression of CD56, IL-2R, CD2, CD11a/CD18,
    ICAM-1, and TNF-R (75 kDa) on NK cells
Inhibits IgE sythesis

Granulocyte-macrophage colony stimulating factor

Granulocyte-macrophage colony stimulating factor (GM-CSF) stimulates the formation of granulocyte, macrophage, mixed granulocyte–macrophage and, at higher concentrations, eosinophil colonies from pluripotent haematopoietic stem cells. It has numerous actions on mature neutrophils, eosinophils, basophils, and macrophages (65; *Table 2.15*). It is produced by a variety of

Table 2.15 Biological properties of granulocyte–macrophage colony stimulating factor

Stimulates granulocytes, macrophages, and eosinophils to proliferate and
  differentiate from bone-marrow progenitors
Activates mature neutrophils and eosinophils (antibody-dependent cellular
  cytotoxicity, phagocytosis, and superoxide generation)
Chemotactic for granulocytes and monocytes
Enhances killing by granulocytes and macrophages
Stimulates macrophages to produce TNF, M-CSF, G-CSF, and IL-1

cells including activated T cells, macrophages, and a number of cell lines (*see Table 1.3*).

Medium in which the HTLV-I-infected T lymphoblast Mo cell line had been grown was used to purify the human protein to homogeneity (66); the resulting glycoprotein had a molecular weight of 22 kDa. On SDS–PAGE the natural protein migrates with an apparent molecular mass of between 14 and 35 kDa, the range being due to variable glycosylation. Human GM-CSF has a single open reading frame coding for a 144 amino acid precursor protein. Seventeen amino acids are cleaved from the amino-terminal end to give a mature 127 amino acid protein (67). The protein is coded for by a single gene on chromosome 5 in humans and 11 in the mouse (*Figure 2.1*). Disulphide bonding between the cysteine residues is important for biological activity since reduction leads to loss of biological activity. Mouse and human GM-CSF have 70% nucleotide homology and 54% amino acid homology but there is no cross-species reactivity.

The α and β chains of the GM-CSF receptor have been cloned (68) and are members of the haematopoietin receptor family (27; *Figure 1.6*) with molecular weights of 80 kDa and 130 kDa, respectively. Binding studies have shown that all cells in the neutrophil, eosinophil, and monocyte series bind GM-CSF whilst lymphoid and erythroid cells are negative. There are a small number of receptors per cell (up to a few hundred).

Granulocyte colony stimulating factor

Granulocyte colony stimulating factor (G-CSF) preferentially stimulates the formation of granulocytic colonies and, at a high concentration, granulocyte–

Table 2.16   Biological activities of granulocyte colony stimulating factor

Stimulates proliferation and differentiation of progenitors committed to granulocyte lineage

Enhances antibody-dependent cytotoxicity, phagocytosis, and superoxide generation by mature granulocytes

Enhances tumour lysis by granulocytes

Chemoattractant for granulocytes and endothelial cells

macrophage colonies from pluripotent haematopoietic stem cells. G-CSF also profoundly affects the function of mature neutrophils causing their activation (69; *Table 2.16*). It is made predominantly by activated monocytes and macrophages but also by other cells of mesodermal origin (*Table 1.3*).

Human G-CSF was purified to homogeneity from the culture supernatants of the human bladder carcinoma cell line 5637 (70). The protein has a molecular weight of 19.6 kDa and a pI of 5.5. The full-length cDNA codes for a protein of 204 amino acids of which the first 30, which are hydrophobic, have been determined as the probable signal sequence (71). *O*-Glycanase treatment of the natural protein reduces the molecular weight from 19.6 to 18.8 kDa, suggesting that there are potential *O*-glycosylation sites through serine or threonine. G-CSF from man and mouse are 73% homologous at the amino acid level and exhibit cross-species biological activity.

Binding studies have shown that all cells of the neutrophilic granulocyte series bind G-CSF. The number of receptors per normal neutrophil increases with maturation to 500–3000 per cell. No binding has been seen to cells of the erythroid, lymphoid, eosinophilic, or megakaryocytic lineages. A small amount of binding has been recorded by normal pro-monocytes and monocytes. Two human cDNAs have been cloned for G-CSF receptors of 759 and 812 amino acids, arising from alternative processing of the same gene product (69). The receptors are members of the haematopoietin receptor family (*Figure 1.6*). Like other receptors these may associate with other polypeptides to give a high affinity receptor capable of signal transduction (27).

Macrophage colony stimulating factor

Macrophage colony stimulating factor (M-CSF) stimulates the formation of macrophage colonies from pluripotent haematopoietic stem cells. Like the other colony stimulating factors it also has effects on the mature counterparts, namely on mature monocytes and macrophages (*Table 2.17*). It is produced principally by macrophages and monocytes.

Human M-CSF, purified to homogeneity from urine, showed a molecular weight of 70–90 kDa comprised of two identical subunits (35–45 kDa). Dissociated subunits are not biologically active. The M-CSF gene consists of many exons covering 22 kb of DNA on chromosome 5 in the human (*Figure 2.1*). At

Table 2.17   Biological activities of macrophage colony stimulating factor

Stimulates proliferation and differentiation of progenitors committed to
  macrophage lineage
Maintains survival and causes differentiation of mature macrophages in culture
Increases Class II MHC and Fc receptor expression
Enhances cytokine production of monocytes and macrophages
Enhances tumouricidal activity of monocytes and macrophages
Enhances microbial killing and antiviral activity of monocytes and macrophages

least two differentially spliced mRNAs are expressed by this gene (72,73). The
RNAs code for protein precursors which are processed to give mature M-CSF
proteins. Thus, a 61 kDa protein is coded for by an mRNA which contains a
sequence for 298 amino acids inserted within the coding sequence of the smaller
(26 kDa) precursor. The two precursors share a common amino-terminal sequence
following removal of a 32 amino acid signal sequence; both are processed at the
carboxy-terminus, are glycosylated and then associate in homodimers to give the
active CSF. At least two natural forms of mature M-CSF exist, a 70–90 kDa
glycoprotein composed of two 35–45 kDa subunits, comprising approximately
223 amino acids, and a 40–50 kDa glycoprotein composed of two 20–25 kDa
subunits of around 145 amino acids. The three-dimensional structure of M-CSF
has been reported (74).

The receptor for M-CSF is coded for by the c-*fms* proto-oncogene (75). The
receptor has an intracellular tyrosine kinase domain which may be involved in
signal transduction and is a member of the immunoglobulin supergene family.
Receptors are found on monocytes and macrophages but not on erythroid,
lymphoid, eosinophilic, or megakaryocytic cells although there may be small
numbers on neutrophils. There are an estimated 3000–15 000 receptors on
macrophages, the number increasing with maturity.

Cytotoxins

Lymphotoxin (LT) is a cytokine released by activated T lymphocytes which is
cytotoxic and cytostatic for some tumour cell lines *in vitro* and causes haemor-
rhagic necrosis of certain tumours *in vivo*. It is also released by certain lymphocyte cell lines. It is closely related to TNF which was first described as a factor in
the serum of mice injected with Bacillus Calmette–Guerin (BCG) and subsequently
challenged with endotoxin, which caused the necrosis of some tumours *in vivo*
and was cytostatic for transformed cell lines *in vitro*. TNF is now known to be
made by activated macrophages and other cells (*Table 1.3*) and to have wide-
ranging pro-inflammatory effects (*Table 2.18*). The amino acid homology and
shared biological properties of these proteins has led to them being renamed
TNF-α (TNF) and TNF-β (LT). However, to avoid confusion the terms TNF
and LT will be used here.

Table 2.18   Biological activities of the cytotoxins

Cytolytic and cytostatic for transformed and virus-infected cells
Protect cells from viral infection
Activate granulocytes and macrophages
Promote bone resorption by osteoclasts
Inhibit collagen synthesis and stimulate breakdown
Induce cytokine secretion e.g. IL-2 and IL-6
Co-stimulate T cell proliferation
Enhance B cell proliferation and immunoglobulin secretion
Activate vascular endothelial cells (induce tissue factor secretion, reduce thrombomodulin secretion, decrease fibrinolytic activity, induce ELAM-1 and ICAM-1 expression)
Promote angiogenesis
Increase eosinophil toxicity for parasites
Stimulate proliferation of fibroblasts
Decrease synthesis of lipoprotein lipase in adipocytes
Stimulate acute-phase protein release by hepatocytes
Enhance Class I MHC expression; minor enhancement of Class II MHC expression
Induce fever

Natural LT has a molecular weight of 60–70 kDa. On SDS–PAGE the major species has a molecular weight of 25 kDa and 5% of the material a molecular weight of 20 kDa (76). The LT codes for a protein of 195 amino acids of which the first 24 residues have characteristics of a signal sequence. The mature protein consists of 171 amino acids (18 664 mol. wt). The difference in molecular weights between the cDNA-encoded and natural protein arises from N-glycosylation of the mature protein. The 25 kDa species has 23 more amino acids than the 20 kDa species (77).

TNF purified from natural sources has a molecular weight of 17 kDa (78). The cDNA predicts a single open reading frame of 233 amino acids of which the first 76 residues are a pre-sequence. The mature protein has a molecular weight of 17 356, close to that predicted by conventional biochemical separation and in agreement with the fact that there were no potential glycosylation sites (79).

A significant homology of 35% is found between LT and TNF at the mature protein level, with numerous conservative amino acid changes on alignment. The secreted forms have relatively hydrophilic amino-termini and significantly hydrophobic carboxy-termini. It is noteworthy that only LT is glycosylated and that only TNF has cysteine residues which form intrachain disulphide bonds. Both genes contain four exons and three introns and are encoded on human chromosome 6 in the MHC with only 1200 base pairs separating the two genes (*Figure 2.1*). The two genes are independently regulated and share little homology in their promoter regions. The close linkage of these genes which are preferentially expressed in different cells on the same chromosome is of particular interest.

The major cells producing TNF are mononuclear phagocytes although other cells such as NK and T cells can produce it (80). Its production is particularly stimulated by LPS but also by other cytokines, viruses, and the cell wall components of mycobacteria. Following stimulation of a cell, TNF is rapidly synthesized and released. LT is produced by T and B lymphocytes in response to stimulation by antigens and mitogens: synthesis and release seem to be somewhat slower than that of TNF.

TNF and LT share usage of common receptors of which there are two, of molecular weight 55 and 75 kDa. The extracellular regions are similar for the two receptors, consisting of four domains with characteristic cysteine residues which are similar to those for the nerve growth factor (NGF) receptor and CD40 and OX40 antigens. In contrast the intracellular domains of the two TNF receptors are entirely unrelated, suggesting differing signalling mechanisms and functions (81). The receptors for TNF are trimers made up of either three 55 or three 75 kDa molecules, the formation of these trimers being driven by the trimeric TNF.

It is apparent that many of the biological activities of TNF and LT are similar to those of IL-1 (10; see *Table 2.3*), and are important in both immunity and inflammation. They act on a very wide range of cellular targets and cause enormous numbers of cellular changes. Interestingly some of these changes are associated with the synthesis of new proteins and others with suppression of protein synthesis. Thus, TNF induces synthesis of cytokines such as IL-1 and Class I MHC antigens but suppresses synthesis of lipoprotein lipase.

Transforming growth factor β family

The transforming growth factor (TGF) β family consists of five gene products, three of which (β_1–β_3) are synthesized in humans with β_1 and β_2 products being the most frequent (82,83). The proteins are released from a latent, biologically inactive precursor. Each subunit combines with another via an interchain disulphide bond to give a biologically active homodimer. TGF-β_1 and -β_2 have recently been crystallized (84).

TGF-β_2 are produced by a wide variety of cell types, particularly platelets and activated macrophages. They are involved in tumour development, extracellular matrix protein synthesis, and immunosuppression and have many diverse stimulatory and inhibitory actions on a wide variety of cells (83) (*Table 2.19*).

Table 2.19   Biological activities of TGF-β

Inhibits the growth of a variety of normal and transformed cells
Mitogenic for some mesenchymal cells e.g. fibroblasts
Promotes extracellular matrix formation
Inhibits proliferation and cytokine release by T cells
Inhibits B cell maturation and proliferation
Inhibits NK activity
Induces bone resorption
Induces integrin expression

There are three structurally distinct receptors for TGF-β (Types I, II, and III). These receptors are complex, possibly reflecting the variable biological effects of the cytokine on different cells, and are widely distributed.

Other cytokines

There are other cytokines which have been cloned and which are undergoing investigation. At the time of writing IL-13 has been described (85); interestingly, this was cloned by screening of a subtracted cDNA library from activated human peripheral blood cells and the activity of the cloned protein was determined. This represents a new and alternative approach to the methods used previously in which the known biological activity was used for purification of a protein, or for isolation of cDNA by expression cloning. Undoubtedly there are many new cytokines to be described, whose genes are determined by a variety of methods. Other cytokines which have been known for longer, like migration inhibition factor (MIF), have been cloned although their detailed real function remains elusive (86). The scope of this book does not permit description of all the cytokines and further details of these can be found from extensive accounts under Further reading.

Further reading

Arai, K. and de Vries, J. E. (1991) *Lymphokines; the molecular biology of regulators of immune and inflammatory responses*. Macmillan, London.

Callard, R. E. and Gearing, A. J. H. (1994) *The cytokine facts book*. Academic Press, London.

De Maeyer, E. and De Maeyer-Guignard, J. (1988) *Interferons and other regulatory cytokines*. John Wiley, New York.

Platzer, E. (1989) Human haemopoietic growth factors. *Eur. J. Haematol.*, **42**, 1.

References

1. Langer, J. A. and Pestka, S. (1985) *Pharmacol. Ther.*, **27**, 371.
2. Langer, J. A. and Pestka, S. (1988) *Immunol. Today*, **9**, 393.
3. Mosmann, T. R. and Coffman, R. L. (1989) *Annu. Rev. Immunol.*, **7**, 145.
4. Naylor, S. L., Sakaguchi, A. Y., Shows, T. B., Law, M. L., Goeddel, D. V., and Gray, P. W. (1983) *J. Exp. Med.*, **157**, 1020.
5. Naylor, S. L., Gray, P. W., and Lalley, P. A. (1984) *Somat. Cell Mol. Genet.*, **10**, 531.
6. Gray, P. W. and Goeddel, D. V. (1982) *Nature*, **298**, 859.
7. Aguet, M., Dembic, Z., and Merlin, G. (1988) *Cell*, **55**, 273.
8. Aguet, M. (1990) *J. Interferon Res.*, **10**, 551.
9. Friedman, R. and Stark, G. (1985) *Nature*, **314**, 637.
10. Dinarello, C. (1991) *Blood*, **77**, 1627.
11. Kimball, E. S., Pickeral, S. F., Oppenheim, J. J., and Rossio, J. L. (1984) *J. Immunol.*, **133**, 256.

12. Dinarello,C.A., Clowes,G.H.A., Gordon,A.H., Saravis,C.A., and Wolff,S.M. (1984) *J. Immunol.*, **133**, 1332.
13. Lomedico,P.T., Gubler,U., and Mizel,S.B. (1987) *Lymphokines*, **13**, 139.
14. Dinarello,C.A. and Wolff,S.M. (1993) *N. Eng. J. Med.*, **328**, 106.
15. Smith,K.A. (ed.) (1988) *Interleukin 2*. Academic Press, San Diego.
16. Holbrook,N.J., Smith,K.A., Fornace,A.J., Comeau,C., Wiskoci,R.L., and Crabtree,G.R. (1984) *Proc. Natl. Acad. Sci. USA*, **81**, 1634.
17. Robb,R.J., Greene,W.C., and Rusk,C.M. (1984) *J. Exp. Med.*, **160**, 1126.
18. Kondo,S., Shimizu,A., Maeda,M., Tagaya,Y., Yodoi,J., and Honjo,T. (1986) *Nature*, **320**, 75.
19. Teshigawara,K., Wang,H.M., Kato,K., and Smith,K.A. (1987). *J. Exp. Med.*, **165**, 223.
20. Takeshita,T., Asao,H., Ohtani,K., Ishii,N., Kumaki,S., Tanaka,N., Munakata,H., Nakamura,M., and Sugamura,K. (1992) *Science*, **257**, 379.
21. Wang,H.M. and Smith,K.A. (1987). *J. Exp. Med.*, **166**, 1055.
22. Cantrell,D.A. and Smith,K.A. (1983) *J. Exp. Med.*, **158**, 1895.
23. Siegel,J.P., Sharon,M., Smith,P.L., and Leonard,W.J. (1987) *Science*, **238**, 75.
24. Shrader,J.W. (ed.) (1988) *Interleukin 3: The panspecific hemopoietin. Lymphokines*, volume 15. Academic Press, New York.
25. Fung,M.C., Hapel,A.J., Ymer,S., Cohen,D.R., Johnson,R.M., Campbell,H.D., and Young,I.G. (1984) *Nature*, **307**, 233.
26. Yang,Y.C., Ciarletta,A.B., Temple,P.A., Chung,M.P., Kovacic,S., Witek-Giannotti,J.S., Leary,A.C., Kriz,R., Donahue,R.E., Wong,G.G., and Clark,S.C. (1986) *Cell*, **47**, 3.
27. Miyajima,A., Kitamura,T., Harada,N., Yokota,T., and Arai,K.-I. (1992) *Annu. Rev. Immunol.*, **10**, 295.
28. Paul,W.E. and Ohara,J. (1987) *Annu. Rev. Immunol.*, **5**, 429.
29. Paul,W.E. (1991) *Blood*, **77**, 1859.
30. Lee,F., Yokota,T., Ostsuka,T., Meyerson,P., Villaret,D., Coffman,R., Mosmann,T., Rennick,D., Roehm,N., Smith,C., Zlotnik,A., and Arai,K. (1986) *Proc. Natl. Acad. Sci. USA*, **83**, 2061.
31. Yokota,T., Otsuka,T., Mosmann,T., Banchereau,J., Defrance,T., Blanchard,D., de Vries,J.E., Lee,F., and Arai,K. (1986) *Proc. Natl. Acad. Sci. USA*, **83**, 5894.
32. Galizzi,J.-P., Zuber,C.E., Harada,N., Gorman,D.M., Djossou,O., Kastelein,R., Banchereau,J., Howard,M., and Miyajima,A. (1990) *Int. Immunol.*, **2**, 669.
33. Sanderson,C.J., Campbell,H.D., and Young,I.G. (1988) *Immunol. Rev.*, **102**, 29.
34. Yokota,T., Arai,N., de Vries,J., Spits,H., Banchereau,J., Zlotnik,A., Rennick,D., Howard,M., Takebe,Y., Miyatake,S., Lee,F., and Arai,K.I. (1988) *Immunol. Rev.*, **102**, 137.
35. Kinashi,T., Harada,N., Severinson,E., Tanabe,T., Sideras,P., Konishi,M., Azuma,C., Tominaga,A., Bergstedt-Lindqvist,S., Takahashi,M., Matsuda,F., Yaoita,Y., Takatsu,K., and Honjo,T. (1986) *Nature*, **324**, 70.
36. Campbell,H.D., Tucker,W.Q., Hort,Y., Martinson,M.E., Mayo,G., Clutterbuck, E.J., Sanderson,C.J., and Young,I.G. (1987) *Proc. Natl. Acad. Sci. USA*, **84**, 6629.
37. Takaki,S., Tominaga,A., Hitoshi,Y., Mita,S., Sonoda,E., Yamaguchi,N., and Takatsu,K. (1990) *EMBO J.*, **9**, 4367.
38. Mita,S., Takaki,S., Hitoshi,Y., Rolink,A.G., Tominaga,A., Yamaguchi,N., and Takatsu,K. (1991) *Int. Immunol.*, **3**, 665.
39. Van Snick,J. (1990) *Annu. Rev. Immunol.*, **8**, 253.
40. Van Damme,J., Opdenakker,G., Simpson,R.J., Rubira,M.R., Cayphas,S., Vink,A., Billiau,A. and Van Snick,J. (1987) *J. Exp. Med.*, **165**, 914.
41. Hirano,T., Yasukawa,K., Harada,H., Taga,T., Watanabe,Y., Matsuda,T., Kashiwamura,S., Nakajima,K., Koyama,K., Iwamatsu,A., Tsunasawa,S., Sakiyama,F., Matsui,H., Takahara,Y., Taniguchi,T., and Kishimoto,T. (1986) *Nature*, **324**, 73.

42. Yamasaki,K., Taga,T., Hirata,Y., Yawata,H., Kawanishi,Y., Seed,B., Taniguchi,T., Hirano,T., and Kishimoto,T. (1988) *Science*, **241**, 825.
43. Taga,T., Hibi,M., Hirata,Y., Yamasaki,K., Yasukawa,K., Matsuda,T., Hirano,T., and Kishimoto,T. (1989) *Cell*, **58**, 573.
44. Henny,C.S. (1989) *Immunol. Today*, **10**, 170.
45. Samaridis,J., Casorati,G., Traunecker,A., Iglesias,A., Gutierrez,J.C., Müller,U., and Palacious,R. (1991) *Eur. J. Immunol.*, **21**, 453.
46. Goodwin,R.G., Lupton,S., Schmierer,A., Hjerrild,K.J., Jerzy,R., Clevenger,W., Gillis,S., Cosman,D., and Namen,A.E. (1989) *Proc. Natl. Acad. Sci. USA*, **86**, 302.
47. Goodwin,R.G., Friend,D., Ziegler,S.F., Jerzy,R., Falk,B.A., Gimpel,S., Cosman,D., Dower,S.K., March,C.J., Namen,A.E., and Park,L.S. (1990) *Cell*, **60**, 941.
48. Sherry,B. and Cerami,A. (1991) *Curr. Opin. Immunol.*, **3**, 56.
49. Oppenheim,J.J., Zachariae,O.C., Mukaida,N., and Matsushima,K. (1991) *Annu. Rev. Immunol.*, **9**, 617.
50. Clore,G.M., Appella,E., Yamada,M., Matsushima,K., and Gronenborn,A.M. (1990) *Biochemistry*, **29**, 1689.
51. Murphy,P.M. and Tiffany,H.L. (1991) *Science*, **253**, 1280.
52. Holmes,W.E., Lee,J., Kuang,W.J., Rice,G.C., and Wood,W.I. (1991) *Science*, **253**, 1278.
53. Van Snick,J., Goethals,A., Renauld,J.-C., Van Roost,E., Uyttenhove,C., Rubira,M.R., Moritz,R.L., and Simpson,R.J. (1989) *J. Exp. Med.*, **169**, 363.
54. Kelleher,K., Bean,K., Clark,S.C., Leung,W.-Y., Yang-Feng,T.L., Chen,J.W., Lin,P.-F., Luo,W., and Yang,Y.-C. (1991) *Blood*, **77**, 1436.
55. Yang,Y.-C., Ricciardi,S., Ciarletta,A., Calvetti,J., Kelleher,K. and Clark,S.C. (1989) *Blood*, **74**, 1880.
56. Fiorentino,D.F., Zlotnick,A., Vieira,P., Mosmann,T.R., Howard,M., Moore,K.W., and O'Garra,A. (1991) *J. Immunol.*, **146**, 3444.
57. Howard,M. and O'Garra,A. (1992) *Immunol. Today*, **13**, 198.
58. Schibler,K.R., Yang,Y.-C., and Christensen,R.D. (1992) *Blood*, **80**, 900.
59. Paul,S.R., Bennett,F., Calvetti,J.A., Kelleher,K., Wood,C.R., O'Hara,R.M.O., Leary,A.C., Sibley,B., Clark,S.C., Williams,D.A., and Yang,Y.-C. (1990) *Proc. Natl. Acad. Sci. USA*, **87**, 7512.
60. Paul,S.R. and Schendel,P. (1990) *Int. J. Cell Cloning*, **10**, 135.
61. Gately,M.K., Desai,B.B., Wolitzky,A.G., Quinn,P.M., Dwyer,C.M., Podalski, F.J., Familletti,P.C., Sinigaglia,F., Chizzonite,R., Gubler,U., and Stern,A.S. (1991) *J. Immunol.*, **147**, 874.
62. Naume,B., Gately,M., and Espevik,T. (1992) *J. Immunol.*, **148**, 2429.
63. Podalski,F.J., Nanduri,V.B., Hulmes,J.D., Pan,Y.-C.E., Levin,W., Danho,W., Chizzonite,R., Gately,M., and Stern,A.S. (1992) *Arch. Biochem. Biophys.*, **294**, 230.
64. Gearing,D. and Cosmann,D. (1991) *Cell*, **69**, 9.
65. Gasson,J.C. (1991) *Blood*, **77**, 1131.
66. Gasson,J.C., Weisbart,R.H., Kaufman,S.E., Clark,S.C., Hewick,R.M., Wong,G.G., and Golde,D.W. (1984) *Science*, **226**, 1339.
67. Wong,G.G., Witek,J.S., Temple,P.A., Wilkens,K.M., Leary,A.C., Luxenburg,D.P., Jones,S.S., Brown,E.L., Kay,R.M., Orr,E.C., Shoemaker,C., Golde, D.W., Kaufman,R.J., Hewick,R.M., Wang,E.A., and Clark,S.C. (1985) *Science*, **228**, 810.
68. Gearing,D.P., King,J.A., Gough,N.M., and Nicola,N.A. (1989) *EMBO J.*, **8**, 3667.
69. Demetri,G.D. and Griffin,J.D. (1991) *Blood*, **78**, 2791.
70. Welte,K., Platzer,E., Lu,L., Gabrilove,J.L., Levi,E., Mertelsmann,R., and Moore,M.A.S. (1985) *Proc. Natl. Acad. Sci. USA*, **82**, 1526.

71. Souza, L. M., Boone, T. C., Gabrilove, J. L., Lai, P. H., Zsebo, K. M., Murdock, D. C., Chazin, V. R., Bruszewski, J., Lu, H., Chen, K. K., Barendt, J., Platzer, E., Moore, M. A. S., Mertelsmann, R., and Welte, K. (1986) *Science*, **232**, 61.
72. Das, S. K., Stanley, E. R., Guilbert, L. J., and Forman, L. W. (1981) *Blood*, **58**, 630.
73. Kawasaki, E. S., Ladner, M. B., Wang, A. M., van Arsdell, J., Warren, M. K., Coyne, M. Y., Schweickart, V. L., Lee, M. T., Wilson, K. J., Boosman, A., Stanley, E. R., Ralph, P., and Mark, D. F. (1985) *Science*, **230**, 291.
74. Pandit, J., Bohm, A., Jancarik, J., Halenbeck, R., Koths, K., and Kim, S.-H. (1992) *Science*, **258**, 1358.
75. Sherr, C. J. (1990) *Blood*, **75**, 1.
76. Aggarwal, B. B., Moffat, B., and Harkins, R. N. (1984) *J. Biol. Chem.*, **259**, 686.
77. Nedwin, G. E., Naylor, S. L., Sakaguchi, A. Y., Smith, D., Jarrett-Nedwin, J., Pennica, D., Goeddel, D. V., and Gray, P. W. (1985) *Nucleic Acids Res.*, **13**, 6361.
78. Aggarwal, B. B., Kohr, W. J., Hass, P. E., Moffat, B., Spencer, S. A., Henzel, W. J., Bringman, T. S., Nedwin, G. E., Goeddel, D. V., and Harkins, R. N. (1985) *J. Biol. Chem.*, **260**, 2345.
79. Pennica, D., Nedwin, G. E., Hayflick, J. S., Seeburg, P. H., Derynck, R., Palladino, M. A., Kohr, W. J., Aggarwal, B. B., and Goeddel, D. V. (1984) *Nature*, **312**, 724.
80. Beutler, B. and Cerami, A. (1989) *Annu. Rev. Immunol.*, **7**, 625.
81. Tartaglia, L. A. and Goeddel, D. V. (1992) *Immunol. Today*, **13**, 151.
82. Massagué, J. (1990) *Annu. Rev. Cell Biol.*, **6**, 597.
83. Bock, M. B. and Marsh, J. (eds) (1991) *Clinical applications of TGF β*. Ciba Foundation Symposium **157**. John Wiley and Sons, Chichester.
84. Daopin, S., Piez, K. A., Ogawa, Y., and Davies, D. R. (1992) *Science*, **257**, 369.
85. Minty, A., Chalon, P., Derocq, J.-M., Dumont, X., Guillemot, J.-C., Kaghad, M., Labit, C., Leplatois, P., Liauzun, P., Miloux, B., Minty, C., Casellas, P., Loison, G., Lupker, J., Shire, D., Ferrara, P., and Caput, D. (1993) *Nature*, **362**, 248.
86. Weiser, W. Y., Temple, T. A., Witek-Giannotti, J. S., Remold, H. G., Clark, C. C., and David, J. R. (1989) *Proc. Natl. Acad. Sci. USA*, **86**, 7522.

3

Cytokines in the activation of T cells, B cells, and macrophages

---

Cytokines in T cell activation, proliferation, and differentiation

The interaction of resting T cells with antigen and cytokines results in their activation, proliferation, and differentiation. The clonal expansion of T cells is dependent on the presence of antigen-presenting accessory cells (APCs) which for CD4$^+$ T cells are usually mononuclear phagocytes or dendritic cells expressing Class II MHC and for CD8$^+$ T cells are any cell expressing Class I MHC. Antigen peptides are presented to the T cell receptor on CD8$^+$ or CD4$^+$ cells in association with Class I and Class II MHC antigens, respectively. In addition to the signals from antigen in association with MHC, signals delivered by cytokines also facilitate T cell activation. Thus, it is generally held that CD4$^+$ cells respond to the dual signals of MHC Class II plus antigen and IL-1 generated by the APCs, although it is not clear that the signal from IL-1 is mandatory. CD8$^+$ T cell responses are augmented by IL-1 and IL-6. Activation of T cells results in the release of other cytokines which affect the growth and differentiation of T cells themselves, B cells, and other cells involved in immune responses. Thus, IFN-γ causes increased class II MHC expression on macrophages as well as their increased IL-1 production in the presence of LPS. Both increased Class II MHC expression and IL-1 production serve to activate T cells further. Additional cytokines made by activated lymphocytes include IL-3, IL-4, IL-5, IL-6, IL-7, IL-10, GM-CSF, TNF-α and -β, and TGF-β.

The types of cytokines released by different subpopulations of CD4$^+$ T cells are thought to influence different facets of the immune response. From studies of cloned T cells in mice there is evidence that there are two subpopulations of CD4$^+$ T cells which secrete different cytokines (1,2; *Table 3.1*). TH1 cells secrete IFN-γ, LT, and IL-2 whereas TH2 cells secrete IL-4, IL-5, IL-6, and IL-10. Both types of cells can secrete IL-3, GM-CSF, and TNF. Studies in bacterial disease (3,4) and allergic disease in humans (5,6) support the differential synthesis

Table 3.1   Different TH cells make different cytokines

	IFN-γ	LT	IL-2	IL-3	IL-4	IL-5	IL-6	IL-10	GM-CSF	TNF
TH1 CD4$^+$	++	++	++	++	−	−	−	−	++	+
TH2 CD4$^+$	−	−	−	++	++	++	++	++	+	+

− None; + Small amounts; + + Large amounts

of cytokines corresponding to the murine cellular profiles. The activities of the cytokines synthesized suggest that the two types of T cells have different functions (*Figure 3.1*). Thus TH1 cells secrete the cytokines associated with cellular immunity, that is the development of delayed hypersensitivity and macrophage activation, whereas TH2 cells secrete cytokines associated with B cell activation, proliferation, and differentiation. Furthermore, the two types of cells seem to regulate each other. IFN-γ secreted by TH1 cells inhibits cytokine production by TH2 cells and IL-10 secreted by TH2 cells inhibits cytokine production by TH1 cells. Preferential activation of one T cell type may explain why immunity in some circumstances appears to be 'cellular' and in others 'humoral'.

The clonal expansion of CD4$^+$ and CD8$^+$ lymphocytes is critically dependent on the generation of IL-2 and IL-2 receptors (IL-2Rs) (7). The major source of IL-2 for proliferation of both these cell types is the CD4$^+$ cell (8). Resting T cells (in G$_0$) are activated by antigen via the T cell receptor to proceed to G$_1$. Here they become responsive to IL-1 and other cytokines and regulatory factors and are induced to synthesize cytokines such as IL-2. Induction of the gene takes around 45 min and is preceded by inositol phospholipid hydrolysis, intracellular Ca^{2+} mobilization, PKC activation, and induction of nuclear transcription factors. The control of IL-2 production rests at the transcriptional level via a 5′ enhancer element (9,10). Following stimulation there is transcriptional activation of the IL-2 gene over 24–48 h. The level of secreted IL-2 corresponds well with the level of intracellular IL-2 mRNA, and this, in turn, depends on the level of transcription and stabilization of message within the cells (11). IL-2 released from the cells binds to the IL-2R to lead to clonal proliferation (*Figure 3.2*).

T cells respond to IL-2 via binding to the high affinity IL-2R made up of the non-covalently linked 55 kDa (α subunit) and 75 kDa (β subunit) chains (12; see Chapter 2). The role of the recently cloned γ chain of the IL-2R is not clear (13). IL-2 can act in an autocrine or paracrine fashion by binding to the intermediate affinity p75 molecule which is constitutively expressed on T cells. This transmits a message to the cell to synthesize the p55 component of the IL-2R and this gives rise to the high affinity IL-2 receptor. Binding of IL-2 to this results in increased Ca^{2+} association with the cells, intracellular alkalinization via activation of the Na$^+$/H$^+$ antiport and via protein tyrosine kinase phosphorylation, although the receptor itself does not have tyrosine kinase activity. Following binding of IL-2 to its receptor, the complex is internalized and therefore removed from the cell surface, and degraded in lysosomes. The half-life at 37 °C for this event is 20–30 min. The induction of the transferrin receptor and progression from G$_1$ to S phase, in which DNA synthesis occurs, follows (14,15).

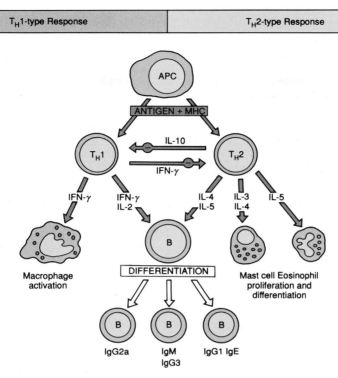

Figure 3.1. Immune responses mediated by TH1 and TH2 cells. TH1 cells produce IFN-γ which activates macrophages and favours B cell differentiation to IgG2a production (in mouse) and inhibits IgG2b and IgG3, thus promoting a cell-mediated immune response. TH2 cells produce IL-3, IL-4, and IL-5 which causes mast cells and eosinophils to proliferate and favours differentiation of B cells to produce IgG1 and IgGE, thereby promoting a humoral type of immune response. Note how IFN-γ from TH1 and IL-10 from TH2 inhibit the actions of the other subpopulation, thus helping to stabilize one pattern of immune response. (In man IL-4 enhances IgG4 and IgE.)

The time course of p55 receptor expression parallels proliferation with both induction and down-regulation playing an important role in controlling the response (16). The number of T cells which become committed to division by passage of the cells from G_1 to S phase of the cell cycle is dictated by the number of occupied IL-2Rs on the cell and thus the concentration of IL-2. The proliferative response to IL-2 thus depends on the occupancy of a critical number of high affinity IL-2Rs and this will depend on the number of receptors, the IL-2 concentration, and the length of the IL-2–IL-2R interaction. Removal of the T cell stimulant results in down-regulation of receptor expression and decline in proliferation, thus limiting the response.

The role of other cytokines is less clear. Thus there is evidence that IL-1 may not be obligatory for the activation of CD4$^+$ T cells (17). T cells have receptors for IL-1 (18) the production of which is initiated by a number of substances

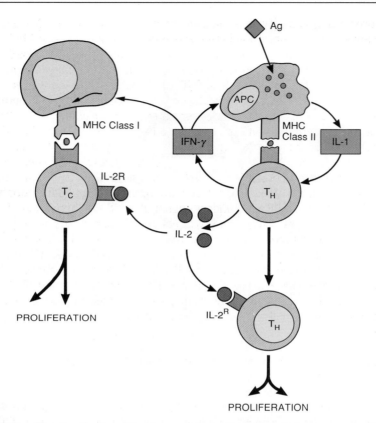

Figure 3.2.   T cell activation. T cells are activated by a signal of processed antigen plus MHC on an APC followed by specific cytokines which drive proliferation and differentiation. IFN-γ from Tн cells can enhance MHC expression and antigen presentation on the APCs. IL-2 is required for proliferation of both Tн and Tc (cytotoxic) cells. IL-1 from macrophages can potentiate activation by increasing IL-2 receptor expression. (Ag = antigen.)

interacting with macrophages/monocytes. Exposure of T cells to IL-1 results in transcription of a number of genes including IL-2, IL-3, and the IL-2R (19). Whether the T cell interacts with soluble IL-1 released from monocytes or a membrane-associated form has not been determined (20). Whilst it was originally believed that IL-1 produced by APCs was an essential component of T cell responses, the current evidence suggests that it has an enhancing rather than obligatory role (17). Thus it has been shown that IL-1 added to T cells rigorously depleted of accessory cells cannot restore the responses to antigen, and that anti-IL-1 antibodies have no effect on T cell proliferation by antigen. Furthermore, dendritic cells which are potent APCs do not produce IL-1, although their antigen-presenting capacity is enhanced by its presence (21). However, IL-1 does enhance T cell proliferation in the presence of low numbers of APCs and IL-1 results in thymocyte proliferation as seen in the bioassay based on this phenomenon. It may be that in the presence of adequate numbers of accessory cells the adhesion between them and T cells via the antigen–Class II MHC interactions may be sufficient. However, in the presence of low numbers of accessory cells, IL-1 is required to optimize the cellular contacts (17,21).

Several other cytokines affect T cells, either on their own (i.e. they are mitogenic) or in the presence of other signals (i.e. they are comitogenic). IL-4 is a growth factor for both CD4$^+$ and CD8$^+$ T cells, although less potent than IL-2 (3,22) and upon interaction with T cells bearing an IL-4 receptor can cause proliferation. IL-6 is involved in T cell activation, growth, and differentiation (23) and like IL-1 can provide a secondary signal after T cell activation. IL-7 also appears to be a cytokine which can provide a second signal to mature peripheral T cells as well as affecting thymocyte maturation (24). IL-12 stimulates the proliferation of activated T cells, and enhances IL-2-dependent proliferation. TNF receptors are induced on activated T cells and, in the presence of TNF, T cells are stimulated to express more receptors for IL-2 and IFN-γ. These examples illustrate the complex interactions of cytokines produced by T cells with both the same T cells, other T cells, B cells, and macrophages.

Cytokines in B cell activation, proliferation, and differentiation

It has been the tradition to consider that the B cell response to antigen occurs in three sequential steps: activation, proliferation, and differentiation. Cytokines which influence B cells were originally divided broadly into B cell activation growth and differentiation factors on the basis of their activity in activation, proliferation, and differentiation assays analysed separately in laboratory experiments (25,26). B cell activation may be examined by looking at the very early events such as changes in phospholipid metabolism, calcium flux, protein phosphorylation, and intracellular pH which occur seconds or minutes after ligand receptor binding. Alternatively, they may be measured by later events such as increase in cell size or expression of activation antigens such as MHC Class II, the IL-2R (CD25) or the low affinity Fcε receptor (CD23) occurring some hours after ligand–receptor interaction. B cell proliferation is measured by incorporation of [^{3}H]thymidine into DNA. In practice this is usually undertaken in co-stimulation assays in which B cells are cultured with a growth factor and a low dose of a polyclonal activator such as anti-IgM or LPS. B cell differentiation is measured as the ability of cells to produce antibody. This may be by incubation of B cells with a differentiation factor and an activation signal and examination of antibody production after some days in culture. Alternatively, B cell lines may be incubated with a differentiation factor and assayed for immunoglobulin production. Finally, differentiation may be assessed from the ability of cytokines to replace TH cells (T cell replacing factors) in antigen-specific antibody responses *in vitro*.

Using these assays, the stages of B cell activation, proliferation, and differentiation have been studied in both human and mouse. In both species it is now clear that the same cytokine may influence all these processes. Other cytokines only seem to operate at one particular stage. Whilst there is broad similarity between human and mouse, there are also some differences; notably, human IL-5 does not seem to be a B-cell growth factor, whereas the cytokine designated as BCGF$_{low}$ does seem to play a role.

A scheme showing the points at which different cytokines act is shown in *Figure 3.3*. From this it is clear that the same cytokine may act at different stages of B cell development —influencing activation, proliferation, and differentiation—and that many different cytokines are involved. The idea of separate growth and differentiation factors is not correct. In addition there is considerable redundancy, with many cytokines having overlapping activities. None of the cytokines act exclusively on

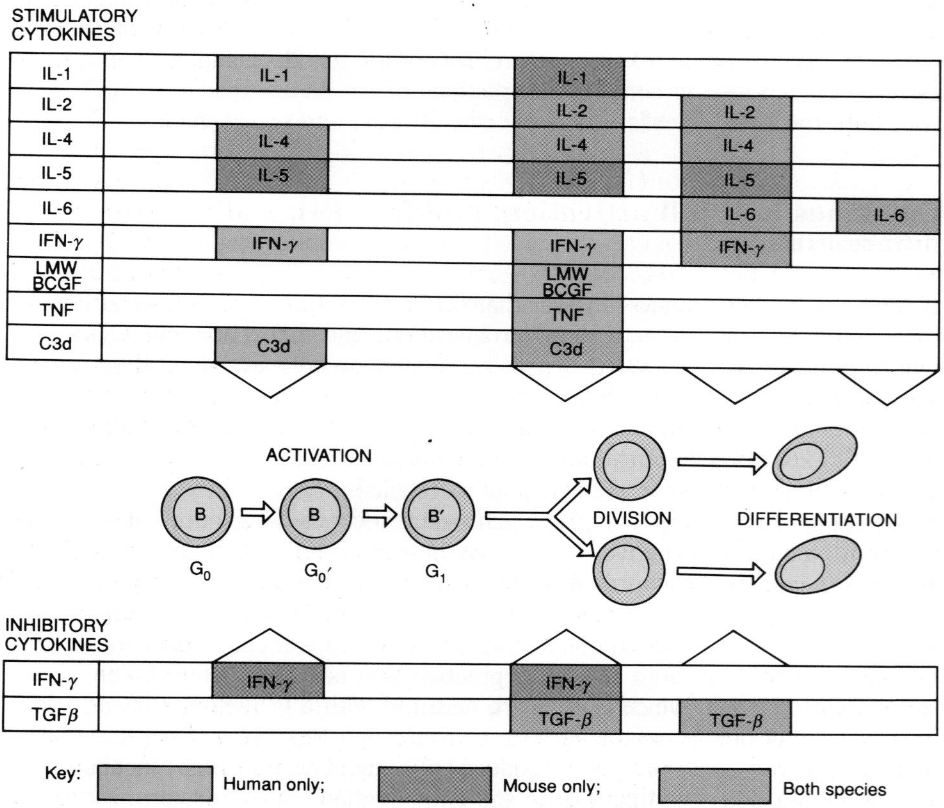

STIMULATORY CYTOKINES

Resting	Activation	Division	Differentiation	
IL-1	IL-1	IL-1		
IL-2		IL-2	IL-2	
IL-4	IL-4	IL-4	IL-4	
IL-5	IL-5	IL-5	IL-5	
IL-6			IL-6	IL-6
IFN-γ	IFN-γ	IFN-γ	IFN-γ	
LMW BCGF		LMW BCGF		
TNF		TNF		
C3d	C3d	C3d		

ACTIVATION

B (G$_0$) ⇨ B (G$_0$′) ⇨ B′ (G$_1$) — DIVISION — DIFFERENTIATION

INHIBITORY CYTOKINES

IFN-γ	IFN-γ	IFN-γ	
TGFβ		TGF-β	TGF-β

Key: ☐ Human only; ▨ Mouse only; ☐ Both species

Figure 3.3. Stages of B cell development. Resting B cells in G$_0$ are activated. The processes of activation, division, and differentiation are modulated by cytokines which can both stimulate or inhibit. LMW = low molecular weight.

cells of the B cell lineage. It may be that different factors act on a different, as yet poorly characterized, subpopulation of B cells. Different antigens may use a different repertoire of B cell factors to produce their final effect and may be responsible for different immunoglobulin isotype production. Finally, it is possible that some of the effects seen are only seen in the specialized cultures used *in vitro*. So far, little is known about the micro-environments *in vivo* where cytokines affecting B cells are generated and exert their action.

The principle cytokines involved in both human and mouse are IL-4 and IL-5 (secreted by TH2 CD4$^+$ cells) and IL-6, although other cytokines have roles as well (1,2). IL-4 enhances class II MHC and FCRε (CD23) expression on resting B cells, co-stimulates proliferation of activated T cells, and stimulates IgE production. IL-5 stimulates proliferation and differentiation and enhances IgA production, and IL-6 induces proliferation and differentiation. Co-stimulators for proliferation and differentiation include IL-1, IL-2, and TNF. In humans the 12 kDa cytokine called BCGF$_{low}$ has been reported to be important in activation and proliferation (27). It has been suggested that BCGF$_{low}$ can cause CD23 to be cleaved to release a soluble product which itself has growth factor activity for B cells (28). IFN-γ inhibits the effects of IL-4 although it has also been reported to have co-stimulatory activities.

Cytokines are involved in the regulation of the isotypes produced by B cells. Activation of B cells *in vitro* in the presence of IL-4 stimulates IgE and IgG1 production in the mouse (1,29) and IgE and IgG4 production in humans (30). *In vivo*, the elevated levels of IgE found in mice infected with *Nippostrongylus brasiliensis* can be inhibited by administration of an anti-IL-4 antibody (31). IL-4-mediated induction of IgE and the elevation seen in *Nippostrongylus*-infected animals can also be inhibited by IFN-γ (32,33). The differences in IL-4 and IFN-γ secretion between TH1 and TH2 CD4$^+$ cells suggest that these two subsets regulate IgE production; such findings have important implications for the development of allergic responses. In addition, IFN-γ has been reported to inhibit IgG1, IgG2b, and IgG3 production but to stimulate IgG2a production (32). In mice IL-5 induces increased production of IgA although this seems to be more in the way of terminal differentiation than isotype switching (34).

In the above descriptions B cell growth and differentiation are depicted as controlled by antigen-driven, T-cell-derived factors augmented by macrophage-derived factors. There is also evidence that B cells have the capacity to control their own growth in an autocrine fashion. Some B cell lines can produce factors such as IL-4 which stimulate their own growth (35) and there is evidence that normal B cells can also respond to factors they make themselves (28). Such autostimulation must be self-limiting if it is not to lead to uncontrolled growth.

The mechanism by which normal B cell responses are regulated is being clarified. However, a number of questions remain. *In vivo* the activation of B cells by T-dependent antigens occurs in lymph nodes in close proximity to the T cells and APCs. In this environment the availability of antigen must limit the response. Presumably, local cytokine and cytokine receptor induction occurs according to the availability of the antigen. Little is known about the control of

TH1 and TH2 cells and the factors which decide the most prominent influence on antibody production. It remains to be seen whether other cytokines are involved. Finally, the way in which cytokines influence antibody production *in vivo* is not well understood. Studies of receptor and cytokine expression within the areas of lymph nodes and other lymphoid organs in which antibody is produced should yield important information with respect to the process and its dynamics.

Cytokines in macrophage activation

Monocytes enter tissues to become resident macrophages which are relatively quiescent cells unless they are stimulated, whereupon they change dramatically. This change, known as macrophage activation, results in increased oxygen consumption, increased functional ability (including phagocytosis and tumour cell killing), changes in cell surface markers (including MHC Class II), and the secretion of numerous biologically active products including cytokines (36). It has long been recognized that T cell activation leads to macrophage activation and it is now appreciated that one of the primary T cell products which has macrophage activating activity is IFN-γ. This cytokine causes increased Class I and Class II MHC expression and increased CR3 expression on macrophages and stimulates

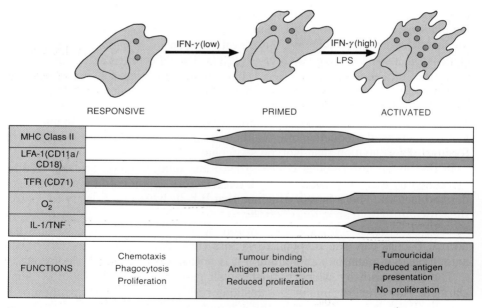

Figure 3.4. Activation of macrophages occurs in two stages. The first is driven by low levels of IFN-γ while the second may be driven by LPS or high levels of IFN-γ. Alterations in the levels of expressed molecules and of cell functions are indicated below. TFR is the transferrin receptor.

these cells to become more active in killing both parasites and tumour cells (32). A model (36) (*Figure 3.4*) suggests that macrophages become fully activated in a two stage process in which they respond first to IFN-γ and then to a second signal of which there are many, although most studies have focused on bacterial LPS. It is probable that priming with IFN-γ is not obligatory for release of all cytokines from macrophages induced by LPS or other substances. However, IFN-γ without doubt amplifies their production. The biologically active products released by activated macrophages include TNF, IL-1, IL-6, GM-CSF, and M-CSF. These in turn exert wide ranging effects on homeostasis of the immune system and immunopathology (see Chapter 4).

Other cytokines can lead to increased macrophage activity. IL-4 increases Class I and Class II MHC antigen expression on human monocytes, up-regulates the expression of CD23, and stimulates the production of G-CSF and M-CSF by macrophages. However, it also inhibits other functions and reduces the expression of other cell surface antigens (*Table 2.5*). GM-CSF and M-CSF are also able to stimulate various aspects of mature macrophage function (*Tables 2.15* and *2.17*). Thus, as for other cells of the immune system, activation of macrophages may result from signals delivered by a number of cytokines. Since different cytokines may be synthesized by different T cell subpopulations, the pattern of macrophage activation may vary accordingly.

Further reading

Callard, R.E. (ed.) (1990) *Cytokines and B cell activation*. Academic Press, London.
Moller, G. (ed.) (1989) T cell activation. *Immunol. Rev.*, **111**.
Oppenheim, J.J. and Shevach, E.M. (eds) (1991) *Immunophysiology: the role of cells and cytokines in immunity and inflammation*. Oxford University Press, Oxford.
Smith, K.A. (1988) *Interleukin 2*. Academic Press, London.

References

1. Coffman, R.L., Seymour, B.W., Lebman, D.A., Hiraki, D.D., Christiansen, J.A., Schrader, B., Cherwinski, H.M., Savelkoul, H.F.J., Finkelman, F.D., Bond, M.W., and Mosmann, T.R. (1988) *Immunol. Rev.*, **102**, 5.
2. Mosmann, T.R. and Coffman, R.L. (1989) *Annu. Rev. Immunol.*, **7**, 145.
3. Yamamura, M., Uyemura, K., Deans, R.J., Weinberg, K., Rea, T.H., Bloom, B.R., and Modlin, R.L. (1991) *Science*, **254**, 277.
4. Salgame, P., Abrams, J.S., Clayberger, C., Goldstein, H., Convit, J., Modlin, R.L., and Bloom, B.R. (1991) *Science*, **254**, 279.
5. Hamid, Q., Azzawi, M., Ying, S., Moqbel, R., Wardlaw, A.J., Corrigan, C.J., Bradley, B., Durham, S.R., Collins, J.V., Jeffery, P.K., Quint, D.J., and Kay, A.B. (1991) *J. Clin. Invest.*, **87**, 1541.
6. Kay, A.B., Ying, S., Varney, V., Gaga, M., Durham, S.R., Moqbel, R., Wardlaw, A.J., and Hamid, Q. (1991) *J. Exp. Med.*, **173**, 775.
7. Robb, R.J. (1984) *Immunol. Today*, **5**, 203.

8. Palacious, H. (1982) *Immunol. Rev.*, **63**, 73.
9. Truneh, A., Albert, F., Golstein, P., and Schmitt-Verhulst, A. (1985) *Nature*, **313**, 318.
10. Weis, A., Wiskocil, R. C., and Stobo, J. D. (1984) *J. Immunol.*, **133**, 123.
11. Ullman, K. S., Northrop, J. P., Verweij, C. L., and Crabtree, G. R. (1990) *Annu. Rev. Immunol.*, **8**, 421.
12. Smith, K. A. (1988) *Science*, **240**, 1169.
13. Takeshita, T., Asao, H., Ohtani, K., Ishii, N., Kumaki, N., Tanaka, N., Munakata, H., Nakamura, M., and Sugamura, K. (1992) *Science*, **257**, 379.
14. Crabtree, G. R. (1989) *Science*, **243**, 355.
15. Cantrell, D. A., Collins, M. K. L., and Crumpton, M. J. (1986) *Immunology*, **65**, 343.
16. Cantrell, D. A. and Smith, K. A. (1984) *Science*, **224**, 1312.
17. Mizel, S. (1987) *Immunol. Today*, **8**, 330.
18. Dower, S. K. and Urdal, D. L. (1987) *Immunol. Today*, **8**, 46.
19. Hagiwara, H., Huang, H. J. S., Arai, N., Herzenberg, L. A., Arai, K. I., and Zlotnick, A. (1987) *J. Immunol.*, **138**, 2514.
20. Kurt-Jones, E. A., Beller, D. I., Mizel, S. B., and Unanue, E. R. (1985) *Proc. Natl. Acad. Sci. USA*, **82**, 1204.
21. Koide, S. L., Inaba, K., and Steinman, R. M. (1987) *J. Exp. Med.*, **165**, 515.
22. Lee, F., Yokota, T., Otsuka, T., Meyerson, P., Villaret, D., Coffman, R., Mosmann, T., Rennick, D., Roehm, N., Smith, C., Zlotnik, A., and Arai, K. (1986) *Proc. Natl. Acad. Sci. USA*, **83**, 2061.
23. Van Snick, J. (1990) *Annu. Rev. Immunol.*, **8**, 253.
24. Morrissey, P. J., Goodwin, R. G., Nordan, R. P., Anderson, D., Grabstein, K. H., Cosman, D., Sims, J., Lupton, S., Acres, R. B., Reed, S. G., Mochizuki, D., Eisenman, J., Conlon, P. J., and Namen, A. E. (1989) *J. Exp. Med.*, **169**, 707.
25. Klaus, G. G. B., Bijsterbosch, M. K., O'Garra, A., Harnett, M. M., and Rigley, K. P. (1987) *Immunol. Rev.*, **99**, 19.
26. Hamblin, A. S. and O'Garra, A. (1987) In *Lymphocytes—A practical approach* (ed. G. G. B. Klaus). IRL Press, Oxford, p. 209.
27. Mehta, S. R., Conrad, D., Sandler, R., Morgan, J., Montagna, R., and Maizel, A. L. (1985) *J. Immunol.*, **135**, 3298.
28. Gordon, J. and Guy, G. R. (1987) *Immunol. Today*, **8**, 339.
29. Vitetta, E. S., Ohara, J., Myers, C. D., Layton, J. E., Krammer, P. H., and Paul, W. E. (1985) *J. Exp. Med.*, **162**, 1726.
30. Lundgren, M., Persson, U., Larsson, P., Magnusson, C., Smith, C. I. E., Hammarstrom, L., and Severinson, E. (1989) *Eur. J. Immunol.*, **19**, 1311.
31. Finkelman, F. D., Katona, I. M., Urban, J. F., Snapper, C. M., Ohara, J., and Paul, W. E. (1986). *Proc. Natl. Acad. Sci. USA*, **83**, 9675.
32. Finkelman, F. D., Holmes, J., Katona, I. M., Urban, J. F., Beckman, M. P., Park, L. S., Schooley, K. A., Coffman, R. L., Mosmann, T. R., and Paul, W. E. (1990) *Annu. Rev. Immunol.*, **8**, 303.
33. de Maeyer, E. and de Maeyer-Guignard, J. (1991) In *The cytokine handbook* (ed. A. Thomson). Chapter 11, p. 215. Academic Press, London.
34. Harriman, G. R., Kunimoto, D. Y., Elliot, J. F., Paetkau, V., and Strober, W. (1988) *J. Immunol.*, **140**, 3033.
35. Blazer, B. A., Sutton, L. M., and Strome, M. (1983) *Cancer Res.*, **45**, 4562.
36. Adams, D. O. and Hamilton, T. A. (1987) *Immunol. Rev.*, **97**, 5.

4

Cytokines in haematopoiesis, cytotoxicity, and inflammation

Introduction

Cytokines are involved in haematopoiesis and the recruitment of cells for host defence. They are important not only for the natural development of white cells during haematopoiesis, but also in the demands for increased numbers of these cells during stress. They are responsible for both the cytotoxic and inflammatory response of a variety of leucocytes to infections and tumours. Produced locally, the effects of the cytokines are restricted by the tissue structure. However, released systemically, they can affect many tissues of the body in a surprisingly large number of different ways. This chapter deals with the role of cytokines in the physiology of the immune system with the emphasis on normal host defence mechanisms, whilst the pathology associated with cytokine release is discussed in Chapter 5.

Haematopoietic cytokines

From *in vitro* data it is believed that a number of cytokines are involved in the maturation and regulated production of blood cells. This has emerged from studies in which single haematopoietic precursor cells from bone marrow, grown in semi-solid culture systems, develop into discrete colonies having recognizable features of mature cells in the presence of growth factors. The CSFs interact with other cytokines at various stages of progenitor cell maturation in a hierarchical fashion (*Figure 4.1*).

Four major CSFs influence haematopoiesis. Two, IL-3 and GM-CSF, have broad specificity, acting on pluripotent stem cells leading to their differentiation, self-renewal, and proliferation (1,2), and two others, G-CSF and M-CSF, act late in haematopoiesis on cells of particular lineages (1–3). In the presence of IL-3, myeloid progenitors are stimulated to develop into many different cell types such

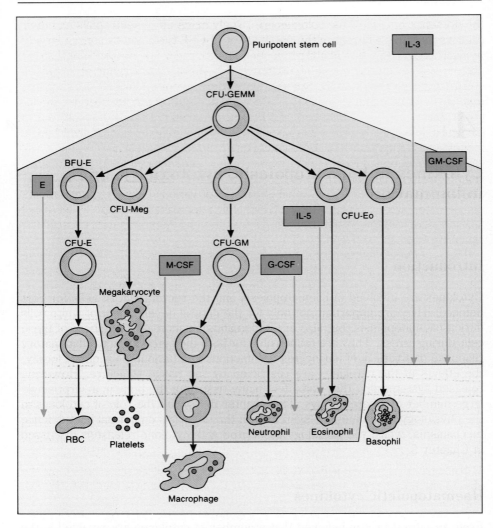

Figure 4.1. Cytokine control of haematopoiesis. The cytokines act in a hierarchical fashion with IL-3 and GM-CSF having wide specificity throughout the differentiation series. M-CSF promotes the macrophage series. G-CSF promotes neutrophils, IL-5 eosinophils, and erythropoietin (E) the differentiation of red blood cells (RBC). (CFU = colony forming unit; BFU = blast forming unit; GEMM = granulocyte, erythrocyte, monocyte, megakaryocyte.)

as early erythrocytes, neutrophils, eosinophils, basophils, macrophages, and megakaryocytes (4–6). GM-CSF gives rise mostly to neutrophils, macrophages, and eosinophils (3). In the presence of erythropoietin and GM-CSF or IL-3, erythrocytes and megakaryocytes develop (2). IL-11 appears to be an additional differentiation factor for megakaryocytes (7), and IL-9 for erythrocytes (8). In the presence of G-CSF the colonies are largely made up of neutrophils and their precursors (4,6), whereas in the presence of M-CSF the colonies consist largely of macrophages (5). Eosinophil production is favoured in the presence of IL-5 (9) and of mast cell production in the presence of IL-4 (10). These findings suggest a stepwise interaction with IL-3 acting on early progenitors which develop into mature cells of multiple lineages, GM-CSF acting somewhat later to similar effect, but G-CSF, M-CSF, IL-4, and IL-5 being committed to actions on cells of particular lineages. Erythropoietin, which is not a cytokine, is produced by the kidney and is important for terminal erythrocyte development and regulation of red cell production (11). Haematopoietin 1, now known to be IL-1, primes stem cells to become responsive to the CSFs (12). IL-2, IL-3, IL-4, IL-5, and IL-6 also exert effects later in the clonal expansion of various cells. Negative effects on haematopoiesis are exerted by TGF-β which decreases the expression of cell surface receptors for growth-signalling molecules and interferes with intracellular signalling from the cell surface (13).

The role these factors play in basal haematopoiesis is unclear. The CSFs have been identified as the products of activated lymphocytes, macrophages, and other cells (see *Table 1.3*). Their source in bone marrow, where maturation normally occurs, is not clear although some are produced by the stromal cells (endothelium, fibroblasts, and perhaps macrophages) of the bone marrow (14).

Many cytokines have also been implicated in the early development of T and B lymphocytes. IL-7, produced by both bone marrow and thymic stromal cells, is important in the proliferation and differentiation of pro-B cells and early thymocytes (15). Additional cytokines produced within the micro-environment of the thymus and the bone marrow seem to play a role in proliferation and differentiation of the cells. In the thymus, IL-1, IL-2, IL-4, IL-6, M-CSF, TNF-α, and IFN-γ have been reported to be produced by various cells and have been implicated in stages of thymocyte maturation. Receptors for these cytokines are similarly present on various cells within the thymus. In the bone marrow, IL-1, IL-3, IL-4, IL-5, and IFN-γ have been implicated (16). TGF-β appears to exert negative effects on lymphocyte maturation in both the bone marrow and the thymus (16,17).

Cytokines play important roles in host defence against infection by recruiting cells, activating them, and ensuring that there are sufficient cells at times of stress. Activated macrophages and T cells produce CSFs directly and IL-1 and TNF can induce other cells such as fibroblasts and endothelial cells to produce GM-CSF (18). IL-5, which is an eosinophil differentiation factor, may be produced by T cell activation during parasite infections and this might lead to the eosinophilia often accompanying these infections (19). By such mechanisms the immune response to an antigen may result in stimulation of bone marrow cells and their release into the blood stream to undertake important functions during infection.

The biological action of the CSFs is not confined to their activity on bone marrow. CSFs released during immune stimulation of peripheral cells can also influence mature cells. Thus GM-CSF activates neutrophils and eosinophils and induces them to undertake antibody-dependent cellular cytotoxicity (ADCC), increase their phagocytosis, and become more adherent (3). It enhances macrophage tumoricidal activity *in vivo* and inhibits neutrophil migration (3). G-CSF stimulates mature neutrophils to undertake ADCC, show enhanced phagocytosis, and produce superoxide in response to f-Met-Leu-Phe bacterial peptide (6,20,21). Thus, factors which are believed to be important in normal haematopoiesis are also involved in the immune response to extrinsic antigens, both by acting back on the bone marrow and by affecting the activity of mature cells.

Cytotoxic and cytostatic cytokines

There are many cytokines which are important in effecting killing of both infectious agents and tumour cells. This killing may be by the direct action of cytokines, as is the case for TNF and LT, or by their indirect action by conferring cytotoxicity on cells or augmenting existing cellular cytotoxicity.

LT was originally identified as a factor from mitogen-activated lymphocytes which had anticellular activity for neoplastic cell lines (22). It is cytostatic for certain tumour lines but has little or no normal anticellular activity. TNF was first described by Carswell as an activity present in serum of mice injected with BCG and subsequently treated with endotoxin (23). It causes necrosis of certain tumours when injected into tumour-bearing animals and is cytotoxic for a number of transformed cell lines *in vitro*. Macrophage cytotoxicity may be mediated by TNF. TNF and LT bind to the same receptor (24) and have the same functional activities. They both cause *in vitro* lysis of actinomycin-D-treated mouse L-929 fibroblasts (25) and necrosis of Meth-A sarcoma tumours *in vivo* (26).

The mechanism by which these substances exert their cytostasis or cytotoxicity is not known. TNF and LT interact with the surface receptors but internalization is required for cell killing. However, many cells that express receptors are not killed, suggesting that something other than receptor–ligand interactions are required for their cytotoxic action. The effects seen in target cells which may contribute to cell death include fragmentation of DNA, the generation of free radicals, and activation of target cell lysosomal enzymes and ADP-ribosylation (27,28). However, at the moment the mechanisms of cytotoxicity and the reasons for the variable sensitivity of different target cells to killing by these cytokines remains unclear (28,29).

In addition to TNF and LT, the IFNs, IL-1, and TGF-β have antiproliferative activity for numerous cell lines (30). TGF-β is a potent inhibitor of normal cell growth including that of endothelial cells, T and B lymphocytes, and NK cells (31). Cytokine production is also down-regulated by TGF-β suggesting an immunoregulatory role for this cytokine (32). However, the effects of TGF-β are reversible and no cell death is seen. Cytokines can act synergistically with each other to enhance cytotoxic/cytostatic effects. Thus, IFN-γ synergizes with LT and TNF in antiproliferative assays *in vitro* (33,34) and, when administered together with LT or TNF, it causes increased antitumour activity. The mechan-

Table 4.1.   Cytokines inducing or augmenting cytotoxicity

Cell	Effect	Cytokines
Macrophages	Activation to kill tumour targets	IFN-γ, IL-2, GM-CSF, IL-4, M-CSF
Polymorphs	Augmentation of antibody-dependent cellular cytotoxicity	TNF, LT, GM-CSF, G-CSF
Cytotoxic T cells	Augmentation of MHC-restricted cellular cytotoxicity	IFN-γ, TNF, IL-12
NK cells and LAK cells	Augmentation of MHC-unrestricted killing	IL-2, IFN-γ, TNF, IL-1, IL-12
Eosinophils	Augmentation of killing of antibody-coated tumour cells	IL-5
Eosinophils	Enhanced toxicity for parasites	TNF, GM-CSF, IFN-γ

isms of this synergy are not understood but it may be that IFN-γ induces more receptors for the cytotoxins on the tumour cells thereby rendering them more susceptible to cytotoxin action, or it may alter the sensitivity of the target cells to the cytolytic mechanisms outlined above.

The generation of new or augmented cytostatic and cytolytic potential in cells exposed to cytokines involves many cytokines and many cell types (*Table 4.1*). Such conferred cytotoxicity may occur on exposure to a cytokine alone or in combination with a second signal, which may be a second cytokine or other stimulant. Amongst these cells, the natural or non-specific MHC unrestricted killer cells have received particular attention (35). These natural killers incubated with cytokines are referred to as lymphokine activated killer (LAK) cells and are capable of greatly augmented killing of tumour cells (36). Their activity has been exploited in therapeutic intervention (see Chapter 5).

Inflammatory cytokines

Cytokines are important in the acute inflammatory response initiated by infection or trauma. The cytokines IL-1, IL-6, and TNF are sometimes referred to as the 'inflammatory triad' since they mediate both local and systemic inflammatory responses which are believed to have survival value (12,28,37,38). IL-1 and TNF are rapidly produced by monocytes and macrophages in response to a number of stimuli such as endotoxin, muramyl dipeptides, lectins, immune complexes, and other noxious agents. Of these bacterial endotoxin has frequently been used both *in vivo* and *in vitro* to stimulate the production of IL-1 and TNF and study their activity. IL-6 is produced by a wide variety of lymphoid and non-lymphoid cells both constitutively and in response to many stimuli including other cytokines. For example, both IL-1 and TNF are potent inducers of IL-6, with IL-1 being 30 times more potent than TNF. Once induced, cytokines may be distributed through the circulation to a larger number of sites of activity. Thus

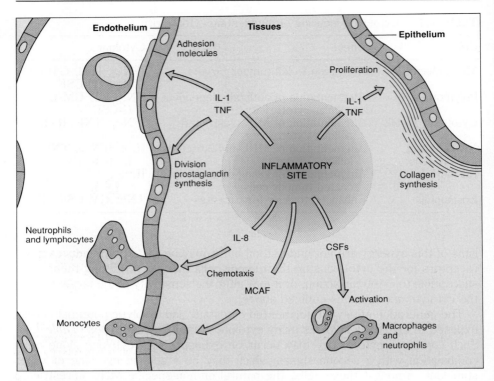

Figure 4.2. Local effects of cytokines in inflammation. IL-1 and TNF act on local endothelium to enhance leucocyte adhesion and migration. IL-8 and MCAF are chemotactic for the migrating cells and CSFs activate phagocytes. IL-1 and TNF also act on epithelium and many mesenchymal cells to cause division and enhance prostaglandin synthesis.

their activity may be represented in both local and systemic inflammatory events (*Figures 4.2* and *4.3*).

The multiple targets and activities of these cytokines are shown in *Tables 2.2, 2.7,* and *2.18*). Locally, IL-1 and TNF induce neutrophil, lymphocyte, and monocyte adherence to endothelial cells, and stimulate endothelial cell procoagulant activity and plasminogen activator inhibitor synthesis. These effects on endothelial cells are important in limiting the spread of infections allowing leucocytes to pass into tissues and accumulate at inflammatory sites. Other local changes brought about by IL-1 and TNF include enzyme release by osteoclasts, chondrocytes, and fibroblasts, and proliferation of epithelial cells, endothelial cells, synovial cells, and fibroblasts. IL-1 induces proteolysis of muscle which releases amino acids for synthesis of new proteins. These activities may have importance in both local inflammation as well as wound healing. In addition IL-1 and TNF produce systemic acute phase changes including neutrophilia, hypozincaemia, hypoferraemia, and increased synthesis of acute phase proteins by

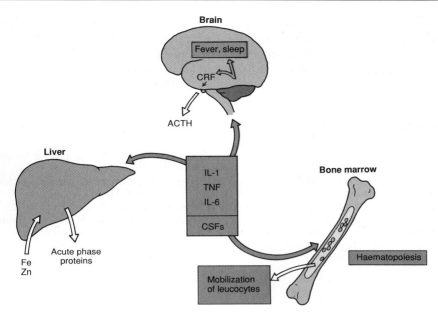

Figure 4.3.   Systemic effects of cytokines in inflammation. The inflammatory triad, IL-1, TNF, and IL-6, act on brain and liver to produce effects beneficial to inflammatory/immune responses. The CSFs may also have long range effects on haematopoiesis and leucocyte mobilization.

hepatocytes. Both also act on the brain to initiate fever, adrenocorticotrophic hormone release, and sleep. These systemic effects are also considered of value in host defence against infection. For example, T and B cell activity are enhanced by fever (39) and release of acute phase proteins and complement assist in the clearance of micro-organisms by the reticuloendothelial system (40). IL-1 and TNF are potent inducers of other cytokines e.g. CSFs, IL-6, IFN-α, and IFN-β, by which means many of their wide range of biological activities may be mediated. Both cytokines are able to induce cells to express many genes but inhibit the expression of others.

Further cytokines implicated in inflammation are IL-8 and the chemokines (41) and the M-, G-, and GM-CSFs (1–6). IL-8 is chemotactic for neutrophils and at higher concentrations for T cells. It induces neutrophil adherence to endothelial cells, the activation of which is implicated in inflammation in which neutrophils predominate (41,42). In a similar fashion MCAF is implicated in inflammatory processes where mononuclear cells predominate (41). As pointed out (Chapter 3) the CSFs are able to activate mature cells and are thus implicated in local activation and recruitment of cells.

Whilst the acute limited production of these cytokines is beneficial, their excessive or sustained production can be deleterious and can result in immunopathology (see Chapter 5). Inflammation is a powerful and protective mechanism by which cells are brought to a site of infection or trauma to clear micro-organisms and effect repair. Cytokines play important roles in orchestrating and controlling the process. However, their continued presence in chronic inflammation or in acute life-threatening inflammation is undesirable.

Further reading

Clark,S.C. and Kamen,R. (1987) The human hematopoitic colony stimulating factors. *Science*, **236**, 1229.

Dexter,T.M., Garland,J.M., and Testa,N.G. (eds) (1990) *Colony stimulating factors; molecular and cellular biology*. Marcel Dekker Inc., New York.

Lord,B.T. and Dexter,T.M. (1992) *Growth factors in haemopoiesis*. Balliere Tindall.

Oppenheim,J.J. and Shevach,E.M. (eds) (1991) *Immunophysiology: The role of cells and cytokines in immunity and inflammation*. Oxford University Press, Oxford.

Sieff,C.A. (1987) Hematopoietic growth factors. *J. Clin. Invest.*, **79**, 1549.

References

1. Schrader,J.W. (1986) *Annu. Rev. Immunol.*, **4**, 205.
2. Sieff,C.A., Emerson,S.G., Donahue,R.E., Nathan,D.G., and Wang,E.A. (1985) *Science*, **230**, 1171.
3. Gasson,J.C. (1991) *Blood*, **77**, 1131.
4. Metcalf,D. and Nicola,N.A. (1983) *J. Cell Physiol.*, **116**, 198.
5. Stanley,E.R. and Heard,P.M. (1977) *J. Biol. Chem.*, **252**, 4305.
6. Demetri,G.D. and Griffin,J.D. (1991) *Blood*, **78**, 2791.
7. Bruno,E., Briddell,R.A., Cooper,R.J., and Hoffman,R. (1991) *Exp. Hematol.*, **19**, 378.
8. Holbrook,S.T., Ohls,R.K., Schibler,K.R., Yang,Y.C., and Christensen,R.D. (1991) *Blood*, **77**, 2129.
9. Clutterbuck,E.J., Hirst,E.M.A., and Sanderson,C.J. (1988) *Blood*, **73**, 1504.
10. Mosmann,T.R., Bond,M.W., Coffman,R.C., Ohara,J., and Paul,W.E. (1986) *Proc. Natl. Acad. Sci. USA*, **83**, 5654.
11. Fisher,J. (1983) *Proc. Soc. Exp. Biol. Med.*, **173**, 289.
12. Dinarello,C.A. (1991) *Blood*, **77**, 1627.
13. Ruscetti,F.W., Dubois,C., Falk,L.A., Jacobsen,S.E., Sung,G., Longo,D.L., Wiltrout,R.H., and Keller,J.R. (1991) In *Clinical applications of TGF-β* (ed. G.R.Bock and J.Marsh). Ciba Foundation Symposium, Vol. 157 p. 227, J. Wiley and Sons, Chichester.
14. Dorshkund,K. (1990) *Annu. Rev. Immunol.*, **8**, 111.
15. Henney,C.S. (1989) *Immunol. Today*, **10**, 170.
16. Carding,S.R., Hayday,A.C., and Bottomly,K. (1991) *Immunol. Today*, **12**, 239.
17. Defrance,T. and Banchereau,J. (1990) In: *Cytokines and B lymphocytes* (ed. R.E.Callard) p. 65, Academic Press, London.
18. Munker,R., Gasson,V.J., Ogawa,M., and Koeffler,H.P. (1986) *Nature*, **323**, 79.
19. Sanderson,C.J., Campbell,H.D., and Young,I.G. (1988) *Immunol. Rev.*, **102**, 29.
20. Platzer,E., Welte,K., Gabrilove,J.L., Paul,L., Harris,P., Mertelsmann,R., and Moore,M.A.S. (1985) *J. Exp. Med.*, **162**, 1788.

21. Lopez,A.F., Williamson,J., Gamble,J.R., Begley,C.G., Harlan,J.M., Klebanoff, S.J., Waltersdorph,A., Wong,G., Clark,S.C., and Vadas,M.A. (1986) *J. Clin. Invest.*, **78**, 1220.
22. Ruddle,N.H. and Waksman,B.H. (1968) *J. Exp. Med.*, **128**, 1267.
23. Carswell,E.A., Old,L.J., Kassel,R.L., Green,S., Fiore,N., and Williamson,B. (1975) *Proc. Natl. Acad. Sci. USA*, **72**, 3666.
24. Aggarwal,B.B., Eessalu,T.E., and Hass,P.E. (1986) *Nature*, **318**, 665.
25. Mathews,N. (1978) *Br. J. Cancer*, **38**, 310.
26. Gray,P.N., Aggarwal,B.B., Benton,C.V., Bringman,T.S., Henzel,W.J., Jarrett, J.A., Leung,D.W., Moffat,B., Ng,P., Svedersky,L.P., Palladino,M.A., and Nedwin,G.E. (1984) *Nature*, **312**, 721.
27. Aggarwal,S., Drysdale,B.E., and Shin,H.S. (1988) *J. Immunol.*, **140**, 4187.
28. Beutler,B. and Cerami,A. (1989) *Annu. Rev. Immunol.*, **7**, 625.
29. Ruddle,N.H. (1987) *Immunol. Today*, **8**, 129.
30. Shalaby,M.R., Hamilton,E.B., Benninger,A.H., and Marafino,B.J. (1985) *J. Interferon Res.*, **5**, 339.
31. Sporn,M.B., Roberts,A.B., Wakefield,L.M., and DeCrombrugghe,B. (1987) *J. Cell Biol.*, **105**, 1039.
32. Chantry,D., Turner,M., Abney,E., and Feldmann,M. (1989) *J. Immunol.*, **142**, 4295.
33. Stone-Wolff,D.S., Yip,Y.K., Kelker,H.C., Lee,J., Henriksen-De Stefano,D., Rubin,B.Y., Rinderknecht,E., Aggarwal,B.B., and Vilcek,J. (1984) *J. Exp. Med.*, **159**, 828.
34. Lee,S.H., Aggarwal,B.B., Rinderknecht,E., Assisi,F., and Chiu,H. (1984) *J. Immunol.*, **133**, 1083.
35. Hersey,P. and Bolhuis,R. (1987) *Immunol. Today*, **8**, 233.
36. Grimm,E.A., Mazumder,A., Zhang,H.Z., and Rosenberg,S.A. (1982) *J. Exp. Med.*, **155**, 1823.
37. Van Snick,J. (1990) *Annu. Rev. Immunol.*, **8**, 253.
38. Oppenheim,J.J., Kovacs,E.J., Matsushima,K., and Duram,S.K. (1986) *Immunol. Today*, **7**, 45.
39. Jampel,H.D., Duff,G.W., Gershon,R.K., Atkins,E., and Duram,S.K. (1983) *J. Exp. Med.*, **157**, 1229.
40. Pepys,M.B. and Baltz,M. (1983) *Adv. Immunol.*, **34**, 141.
41. Oppenheim,J.J., Zachariae,O.C., Mukaida,N., and Matsushima,K. (1991) *Annu. Rev. Immunol.*, **9**, 617.
42. Rampart,M., Van Damme,J., Zonnekeyn,L., and Herman,A.G. (1989) *Am. J. Pathol.*, **135**, 21.

5

Cytokines in pathology and therapy

Since cytokines are important in the regulation of immune responses it follows that their over- or under-production may be involved in the pathology of diseases which directly or indirectly involve the immune system. Furthermore, their potent ability to affect immune cells and their availability in recombinant form provides the rationale and means for their use in immunotherapy. In this chapter the role of cytokines in disease pathology and therapy are considered.

Cytokines and pathology

Cytokines are generally induced rather than constitutively produced. Thus their presence in tissues is indicative of immunological activity. There are many reports that production of cytokines, expression of cytokine genes, cellular expression of cytokine receptors, and release of soluble cytokines receptors are seen abnormally in different diseases. In normal inflammatory processes they are produced in response to stimulation, and after withdrawal of the stimulus production stops. For reasons which often have yet to be understood their production can become sustained and is then associated with the tissue damage seen in acute and chronic inflammatory diseases. In addition, since they play an important part in immune responses to extrinsic antigens, they are likely to be involved in responses to auto-antigens. Finally, since cytokines are growth factors for cells of the immune system it might be expected that they may be involved in the disregulated growth of lymphoid and myeloid tumours.

IL-1, TNF, and IL-6 (the 'inflammatory triad') have been found in elevated levels in the affected tissues of a number of chronic inflammatory diseases. For example, TNF has been found in the joints of patients with rheumatoid arthritis (1), in the brain lesions of patients with multiple sclerosis (2), and in the cells of the affected gut in inflammatory bowel disease (3). Additional cytokines may also be present suggesting disturbance of the cytokine network. Thus, in rheumatoid arthritis elevated levels of GM-CSF and IL-8 as well as TNF, IL-1, and IL-6 have all been reported in affected joints (4).

65

The systemic effects of cytokines are also important in the inflammatory response accompanying many diseases. There are many examples of diseases in which cytokines such as IL-1, IL-2, IL-5, IL-6, and TNF and soluble cytokine receptors such as those for IL-2, IL-4, IL-7, TNF, and IFN-γ are found in serum. For example, serum IL-5 is found in patients with episodic angioedema and eosinophilia (5) and soluble IL-2 receptor (CD25) is found in the serum of haemophilia patients infected with HIV (6). Since cytokines and soluble cytokine receptors are either absent or present at low levels in normal serum their presence indicates activation either of circulating cells or of cells in tissues resulting in leakage into the blood. In moderation and for short duration these may not be harmful to the host and may be part of the normal inflammatory response (see Chapter 4). However, uncontrolled production may be very damaging. It has been known for a long time that Gram-negative bacterial infection may lead to endotoxic shock (toxic shock syndrome) characterized by, for example, fever, metabolic acidosis, diarrhoea, hypotension and disseminated intravascular coagulation (7). There are a number of strands of evidence that support the view that bacterial endotoxins induce these systemic toxic effects by stimulating the production of IL-1, IL-6, IL-8, and particularly TNF (8). After injection of endotoxin into animals, large amounts of TNF appear in the circulation within minutes, peaking 1–2 h later (9) and injection of recombinant TNF into animals produces endotoxic shock (10). Administration of anti-TNF antibody has been shown to be effective in preventing septic shock in animal models of sepsis (11). IL-6 and TNF have been detected in the serum of toxic shock patients with TNF being found in particularly high levels. Injection of TNF into normal volunteers induces a neutropaenia followed by a neutrophilia, neutrophil and monocyte activation, and a rise in serum IL-6 but not IL-1 (12).

A further deleterious systemic effect of cytokines is the wasting or cachexia associated with cancer and infectious disease. Here, TNF, which is also called cachectin, is believed to be responsible (8,13). It depresses lipoprotein lipase production and this prevents the uptake of exogenous triglyceride and hydrolysis to free fatty acids and glycerol (14). Rodents implanted with tumours continuously secreting TNF from a transfected human TNF gene become wasted (15) (*Figure 5.1*) and infusion of TNF into animals causes anorexia. Thus, it seems that TNF can produce cachexia, although it is not clear how this condition is generated in diseases such as cancer. Some tumour cells themselves have been shown to synthesize TNF, or may stimulate macrophages to do so. In infectious diseases, overwhelming continuous stimulation of macrophages may lead to generation of sufficient TNF to result in cachexia.

Production of cytokines may well produce some of the pathological effects associated with infectious diseases. In acute viral infections such as influenza and measles, interferons may be detected in the circulation and their presence is associated with fevers, chills, and general malaise (16,17). In mice infected with malaria high levels of serum TNF are associated with lethal outcome and particularly with neurological symptoms (cerebral malaria) (18). Administration of anti-TNF reduces the disease symptoms, and antibodies to IFN-γ, and to IL-3 and

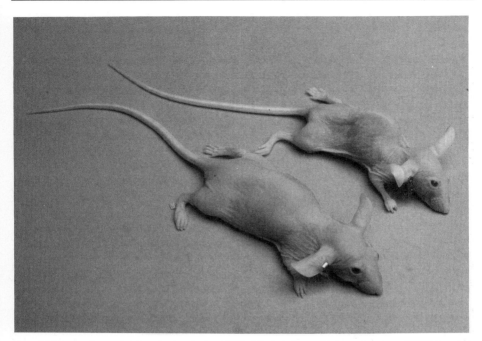

Figure 5.1. Induction of cachexia by TNF. Nude mice which were given CHO tumour cells containing the TNF gene insert are severely wasted (right) by comparison with animals which have the same tumour cells lacking the TNF gene (left). By courtesy of Dr A. Oliff, reprinted by permission of *Cell* (15). Copyright is held by Cell Press.

GM-CSF also modify the disease suggesting that they are involved in a cytokine cascade which influences the outcome (19,20). Since IFN-γ induces macrophages to produce TNF and GM-CSF, and since IL-3 increases the production of monocytic cells from the bone marrow, this may explain why antibodies to these cytokines can modify the disease. In human cerebral malaria very large amounts of TNF are also found in the circulation and again may be responsible for the traumatic effects of this disease.

There is interest in the possibility that imbalances in the proportions and activity of TH1 and TH2 cells may be important in the development of pathology (21). In asthmatics it has been shown by *in situ* hybridization that lymphocytes in the lung contain mRNA for IL-5 (22) and that mRNAs for IL-3, IL-5, and GM-CSF but not for IFN-γ and IL-2, were found in the allergen-induced late-phase cutaneous reactions in atopic subjects (23) suggesting a selective activation of TH2 type cells (*Figure 5.2*). In parasitic diseases there is evidence that different patterns of cytokine release (corresponding to the profiles made by TH1 and TH2 cells) are seen in animals showing different responses to the parasites (24). Infection of most strains of mice with *Leishmania major* leads to a localized cutaneous lesion that heals spontaneously and confers resistance to reinfection. However, in some strains of mice, e.g. BALB/c, the infection progresses to a

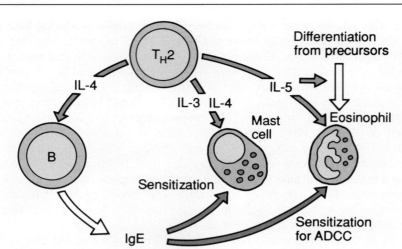

Figure 5.2.   Role of TH2 cells in atopy. TH2 cells promote IgE synthesis by B cells and activate mast cells and eosinophils which are prominent in allergic reactions.

disseminated visceral disease that is usually fatal. Self-healing disease is accompanied by delayed-type hypersensitivity (DTH) and poor antibody responses, whereas non-healing disease is accompanied by strong antibody responses including high IgE levels and little DTH. Evidence exists that the CD4$^+$ T cells from the non-healing animals contain significant levels of IL-4 mRNA but not IFN-γ mRNA whereas the healing mice have cells with substantial levels of IFN-γ mRNA but not IL-4 mRNA (25). The T cells from healing and non-healing infected animals produce either TH1 or TH2 cytokines respectively when stimulated *in vitro* (26), and T cell lines which are of TH1 or TH2 type transfer protection or exacerbation, respectively (27). In humans there is also evidence for differential cytokine expression in disease. In the 'tuberculoid' form of leprosy there are few bacilli present and mRNAs for IL-2 and IFN-γ are most prominent in skin lesions. By contrast, in the multibacillary form, IL-4, IL-5, and IL-10 are most prominent (28). Cloned T cells from tuberculoid and multibacillary patients also produced the different cytokine profiles corresponding to TH1 and TH2 cells, respectively (29). All these findings support the notion that TH1 or TH2 patterns of cytokine release may be associated with pathological outcome in particular diseases. Furthermore, in these situations it is believed that cytokine production by each subset can inhibit the activity of the other, leading to stabilization of either a TH1 or TH2 type of response. Thus, IFN-γ produced by TH1 cells inhibits the activity of TH2 cells and IL-10 produced by TH2 cells inhibits the activity of TH1 cells (cross-regulation, 21). It follows that manipulation of these events may allow prevention of harmful pathology (see below).

Cytokines have been implicated in the development of autoimmunity (1,4). Presentation of auto-antigens may occur when cells which normally do not express Class II MHC products are induced to do so (30,31). Thyrocytes from patients with auto-immune thyroid disease (32) and insulin-producing beta cells in the 'diabetic' pancreas (33) express Class II MHC products, whereas their normal counterparts do not. These cells may bypass the need for normal antigen-presenting cells, and be able to present self-antigens to T cells (34). Activated T cells would then be clonally expanded, become effector T cells, and induce auto-antibody production by B cells. These processes would involve the cytokines important in normal T and B cell activation (Chapter 3). In this model the induction of Class II MHC molecules is critical to the development of auto-immunity. Since IFN-γ is a potent inducer of these molecules, inappropriate production of this cytokine would lead to Class II MHC expression. This might occur as a result of viral infections, which have been implicated in the induction of some endocrine auto-immune diseases (35). The model implies that cytokine production in the wrong place at the wrong time might allow an auto-immune response to emerge with subsequent damaging consequences.

It is an attractive hypothesis that cytokines are involved in the disregulated growth of lymphoid or myeloid cells resulting in leukaemias and lymphomas. Since cytokines can act in an autocrine fashion, it is conceivable that leukaemic cells may emerge because they both produce and respond to growth factors in an uncontrolled fashion. Alternatively, they may grow because they have lost their regulated control by cytokines. For most B and T cell leukaemias and lymphomas, however, there is little evidence of autocrine cytokine regulation, although IL-6 appears to be a growth factor for human multiple myeloma cells (36), IL-2 for some adult T cell leukaemias (37), IL-1β for some acute myelogenous leukaemias (38), and IL-9 for some cases of Hodgkin's lymphoma and large cell anaplastic lymphoma (39).

One mechanism by which disregulated cytokine production may occur is by the insertion of a retrovirus near a cytokine gene leading to increased cytokine production and thus pathology. The WEH1-3B cell line, which produces a myelo-monocytic leukaemia in mice, is also a constitutive producer of IL-3 *in vitro*. It has been shown that there is a 5 kb insert 5′ to the gene which is a type of endogenous murine retrovirus (40) and that this insertion leads to up-regulated expression of IL-3. Retroviral insertion at sites distant from cytokine genes may also affect cytokine production or responsiveness. Infection of both CD4$^+$ T cells and monocytes with HIV leads to disregulated cytokine production which may contribute to the disease pathology. Most T cells infected with the retrovirus HTLV-1, the agent responsible for adult T cell leukaemia, grow *in vitro* without the addition of exogenous IL-2 and constitutively express the IL-2 receptor (41) suggesting that cell growth is dependent on the constitutive production and autocrine action of IL-2. However, the cells not only fail to produce IL-2 constitutively but also cannot be induced to produce IL-2 upon stimulation. In contrast, the IFN-γ gene is both active and inducible suggesting that HTLV-1 does not cause generalized repression of gene expression. Rather it seems that cell growth without IL-2 control may be the very reason for their establishment as leukaemic cells.

There are to date only rare examples of human immunodeficiencies in which a cytokine is not produced, as might occur if there was mutation, deletion, or complete suppression of a cytokine gene. It is of interest that many of the genes for cytokines are located on chromosome 5 and that deletions on the long arm of chromosome 5 are frequently observed in patients with myelodysplastic syndrome, acute non-lymphocytic leukaemia secondary to cytotoxic therapy, as well as refractory anaemia characterized as a '5q-syndrome' (42). However, a causal relationship between the deletion of part of chromosome 5 and these diseases has not been established. It has been shown that the mutation in mice recessive for the osteopetrosis gene, which have a restricted capacity for bone remodelling and are deficient in mature macrophages and osteoclasts, is in the M-CSF gene (43). This shows that mutation in a cytokine gene can be associated with pathology, and is in accord with data from gene-deleted mice, who also often show severe pathology.

It is interesting to speculate on the effect of deletion of a cytokine gene on the survival of the individual. Would other genes coding for cytokines with similar activities compensate for the loss or would the deletion be lethal? Some insight into this is available from current animal studies in which genes are deleted (44; see Chapter 1) and suggest some surprising results (45). Similarly, it is pertinent to ask whether mutation or deletion of a cytokine receptor gene leads to immunodeficiency. The answers to these questions await further studies.

Cytokines and therapy

The interest in cytokines and therapy arises both from their potential direct use as well as from the need to inhibit their production or action. The evidence that they are involved in chronic inflammation (46) has resulted in a burgeoning interest in both synthetic and natural inhibitors (47,48) including cytokine receptors (49). However, since the same mediators implicated in pathology also regulate normal immune responses, it will be necessary to influence abnormal cytokine production and action without damaging normal immunoregulatory networks.

Direct therapy with cytokines has a number of applications. Firstly, cytokines may be used to reconstitute a failed immune system or to recruit cells needed to overcome temporary immunodeficiency such as that following cytotoxic therapy for treatment of tumours or bone-marrow transplantation. Secondly, cytokines may also be used to stimulate the host immune response to tumours or overwhelming infections. In all these areas there is considerable work using recombinant cytokines in both experimental models in animals and clinical studies in humans.

Cytokines which affect haematopoiesis have considerable clinical potential in acute regeneration of myeloid cells after cytotoxic treatment, bone-marrow transplantation, aplastic anaemia, agranulocytosis (idiopathic, toxic, or genetic), congenital or acquired neutrophil dysfunction, and infections (50). Injection of cytokines into both normal and diseased recipients results in the rapid appearance of cells in the blood and tissues. Injection of human recombinant GM-CSF into monkeys (*Macaca fasicularis* or *Macaca mulata*) gave a dramatic dose-dependent leucocytosis, consisting largely of neutrophils, within 24–48 h (51) (*Figure 5.3*). This was maintained for up to 1 month by continuous infusion without substantial side effects. Upon termination of infusion the leucocyte numbers returned to normal in 3–7 days. Administration of GM-CSF to monkeys rendered pancytopaenic with a simian type D retrovirus (51) and monkeys recovering from autologous bone-marrow transplantation (52) showed similar effects. In all cases the elevation was transient and dependent on continuous infusion of the GM-CSF. Similar studies of G-CSF in animals (53) have resulted in this cytokine and GM-CSF being used to accelerate neutrophil recovery after chemotherapy for malignant disease including that used alongside bone-marrow transplantation (50,54,55). These CSFs have been valuable in the treatment of patients with severe congenital neutropaenias, myeloid leukaemia, and myelody-splastic syndromes and are starting to be used for the treatment of severe bacterial, fungal, and protozoal infections (50,54,55). These early successes are being followed by assessment of other cytokines for their ability to stimulate stem cell activity and the rapid regeneration of cells in the circulation.

The application of cytokines to stimulation of immune responses has mostly

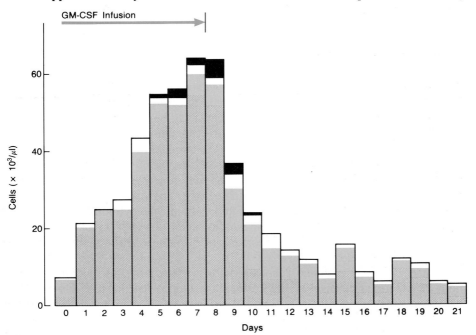

Figure 5.3. Effect of GM-CSF *in vivo*. Normal monkeys were infused with 500 units of human recombinant GM-CSF min^{-1} kg^{-1} for 1 week. Blood counts show a massive increase in neutrophils (grey) and monocytes (white) and pronounced eosinophilia (black) at 4–9 days. Lymphocytes (orange) are also increased, but to a lesser extent. Data of Donahue *et al.*, ref. 51.

been evaluated in patients with tumours. The finding that leucocytes incubated with IL-2 gave rise to a cytotoxic cell capable of killing tumour cells but not normal cells (56) prompted both laboratory investigation and application to human tumour therapy. LAK cells have been shown to be effective in mediating regression of lung and liver metastases in various murine models (57). Although IL-2 alone in very large amounts was shown to affect these tumours, the injection of IL-2 with LAK cells proved to be the most beneficial. Laboratory studies led to clinical trials in which LAK cells were administered with IL-2 in humans (58). Patients' leucocytes were incubated *ex vivo* with IL-2 and then readministered with IL-2. Significant tumour regressions were reported (*Figure 5.4*) although there was also significant toxicity associated with the treatment. The IL-2 gave rise to leaky capillaries and this resulted in fluid retention which caused dose-limiting toxicity. Much of the toxicity probably arose from the induction of other cytokines such as TNF which produced systemic pathology (see above). Of the tumours which regressed, the most significant and long lasting changes were seen for renal cell carcinoma and melanoma. IL-2 or IL-2 and LAK cells seem to show consistent benefit in 10–20% of patients with these two tumours (see Smith *et al.* in Further reading).

Other potential agents for tumour therapy are the interferons IFN-α and IFN-γ, and TNF and lymphotoxin (LT). IFN-γ is immunomodulatory and has been shown to cause macrophage activation in clinical trials (59) but has not shown consistent activity in any malignancies although trials continue. In contrast, IFN-α has been reported to be effective in treating hairy cell leukaemia (60), Kaposi's sarcoma (61), chronic myeloid leukaemia (62), and myeloma (63). TNF has also been studied and although extremely toxic when administered systemically, local administration by perfusion of isolated limbs affected by melanoma and in the treatment of the ascites of ovarian carcinoma may be effective (64).

In these therapeutic manipulations, where the aim is to restore or activate a deficient immune system, it is possible that administration of more than one cytokine may be of benefit. Furthermore, because of the synergistic actions of cytokines, low doses of individual cytokines may together be much more effective than each cytokine on its own. An alternative approach is to create a fusion protein with the active component of more than one cytokine, as has been created for IL-3 and GM-CSF (65). In addition such 'designer' cytokines may find a place in therapy if they limit the toxicity of cytokines whilst at the same time remaining efficacious.

Stimulation of the immune response with cytokines has application to treatment of infectious diseases. There is some evidence that local IFN-γ and IL-2 may have a beneficial effect in lepromatous leprosy, by causing both enhanced immunological responses and some reduction in *Mycobacterium leprae* burden and in cutaneous leishmaniasis (66,67). These effects may result from activation of antimicrobial cells and/or by altering the balance of TH1 and TH2 cells (21).

As an alternative to using cytokines, either to boost the immune response or to substitute for a deficient one, opportunities to manipulate their activities are posed by a number of diseases where their excessive production is believed to

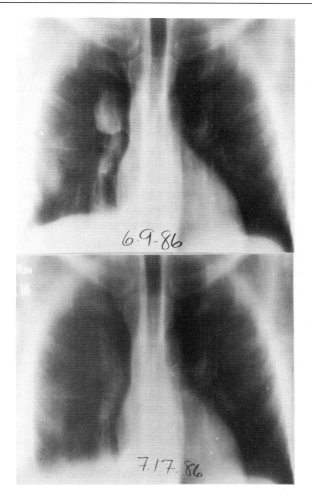

Figure 5.4.   Linear tomograms of lung lesions of a metastatic melanoma before (top) and after (bottom) treatment with a combination of IL-2 and LAK cells. The parenchymal and mediastinal lesion on the left of the top figure regressed appreciably after therapy. By courtesy of Dr S.Rosenberg, reprinted by permission of *The New England Journal of Medicine* (58).

lead to immunopathology. Here monoclonal antibodies against cytokines, or specific inhibitors such as IL-1 receptor antagonist protein (IRAP) (68), or soluble cytokine receptors may be effective (47–49). Thus, antibodies to TNF are being used in the treatment of toxic shock syndrome and are being considered in the treatment of graft versus host disease and rheumatoid arthritis. Antibodies or soluble receptors or agonists for cytokines such as TNF and IL-1 are showing experimental promise and entering clinical trials. In situations where there may be imbalances in the activity of TH1 and TH2 T cell subsets, administration of antibodies or inhibitors may redress this balance. Mice infected with *Nipostrongylus brasiliensis* or *Schistosoma mansonii* produce large amounts of IL-10 but have suppressed IFN-γ production which can be restored with anti-IL-10 antibodies (69). Alternatively, administration of IFN-γ may counter the activity of TH2 cells and IL-10 may counter the activity of TH1 cells. Inhibitory cytokines such as TGF-β offer further opportunities to manipulate cytokine pathways (70).

Some of these approaches are now being used clinically whilst others are only at the experimental or theoretical stages. Any clinical use is preceded by a long process of testing for toxicity and efficiency and it is clear that therapeutic manipulation of cytokine pathways is not without its problems. High levels or repeated doses often lead to side effects which resemble severe influenza. More severe side effects can lead to damage to vital organs. Probably these arise because administration of cytokines induces other cytokines which cause toxicity. The half-life of cytokines is only minutes in the circulation and so therapeutic benefit is only likely to be achieved when the effects cytokines produce can be achieved by short, intense therapy or by the maintenance of sufficiently high levels without severe toxicity or by modifying delivery systems so that cytokines may be targeted to the site at which they are needed. Since cytokines work together, both synergistically and in cascades, it is possible that 'cocktails' of them may produce greater benefit than a single factor. Administration of inhibitors may imbalance the normal cytokine networks in a way which may be deleterious to the host if given for too long. It is therefore likely that these approaches may be most beneficial in short bursts rather than over prolonged periods. Mouse monoclonal antibodies to cytokines will have limited usage in treating human disease because they may invoke an anti-mouse response. 'Humanization' (where the antigen binding site of a mouse antibody of interest is genetically engineered into the framework of a human immunoglobulin molecule) of the monoclonal antibodies may circumvent this problem and it is possible that a short course of antibody may be sufficient to reverse the pathological process.

The clinical value of cytokines has to be carefully evaluated since these are both potent and costly. In spite of much activity, the process of determining safe and effective use of cytokines and their inhibitors for treatment of disease is still at early stages. Many beneficial effects have been found and many interesting possibilities are opening up. It will be some time before the full impact and appropriateness of their use in different clinical situations is fully realized.

Further reading

Metcalf,D. (1989) Haemopoietic growth factors 2: Clinical applications. *Lancet*, **i**, 885.

Oppenheim,J., Rossio,J., and Gearing,A. (eds) (1993) *Clinical applications of cytokines.* Oxford University Press, Oxford.

Romagnani,S. (1992) Human TH1 and TH2 subsets: regulation of differentiation and role in protection and immunopathology. *Int. Arch. Allergy Immunol.*, **98**, 279.

Smith,J.W., Urba,W.J., Steis,R.G., Sznol,M., Creekmore,S.P., and Longo,D.L. (1991)

Clinical trials of selected interleukins; the biological response modifiers programme experience. In *Cytokine interactions and control* (ed. A.Baxter and R.Ross). John Wiley and Sons, Chichester.

References

1. Brennan,F.M., Chantry,D., Jackson,A., Maini,R.N., and Feldmann,M. (1989) *Lancet*, **ii**, 244.
2. Selmaj,K., Raine,C.S., Cannella,B., and Brosnan,C.F. (1991) *J. Clin. Invest.*, **87**, 949.
3. Macdonald,T.T., Hutchings,P., Choy,M.Y., Murch,S., and Cooke,A. (1990) *Clin. Exp. Immunol.*, **81**, 301.
4. Feldmann,M., Brenan,F.M., Chantry,D., Haworth,C., Turner,M., Katsikis,P., Londei,M., Abney,E., Buchan,G., Barrett,K., Corcoran,A., Kissonerghis,M., Zheng,R., Grubeck-Loebenstein,B., Barkley,D., Chu,C.Q., Field,M., and Maini,R.N. (1991) *Immunol. Rev.*, **119**, 105.
5. Butterfield,J.H., Leiferman,K.M., Abrams,J., Silver,J.E., Bower,J., Gonchoroff, N., and Gleich,G.J. (1992) *Blood*, **79**, 688.
6. Noronha,I.L., Daniel,V., Shimpf,K., and Opelz,G. (1992) *Clin. Exp. Immunol.*, **87**, 287.
7. Nishijima,H., Weil,M.H., Shubin,H., and Cavanilles,J. (1973) *Medicine*, **52**, 287.
8. Vassali,P. (1992) *Annu. Rev. Immunol.*, **10**, 411.
9. Beutler,B., Milsark,I.W., and Cerami,A. (1985) *J. Immunol.*, **135**, 3972.
10. Tracey,K.J., Beutler,B., Lowry,S.F., Merryweather,J., Wolpe,S., Milsark,I.W., Hariri,R.J., Fahey,T.J., Zentella,A., Albert,J.D., Shires,G.T., and Cerami,A. (1986) *Science*, **234**, 470.
11. Silva,A.T., Bayston,K.F., and Cohen,J. (1990) *J. Infect. Dis.*, **162**, 421.
12. van der Poll,T., van Deventer,S.J.H., Hack,C.E., Wolbink,G., Aarden,L.A., Buller,H.R., and ten Cate,J.W. (1992) *Blood*, **79**, 693.
13. Beutler,B. and Cerami,A. (1989) *Annu. Rev. Immunol.*, **7**, 625.
14. Mahoney,J.R., Beutler,B.A., Le Trang,N., Vine,W., Ikeda,Y., Kawakami,M., and Cerami,A. (1985) *J. Immunol.*, **134**, 1673.
15. Oliff,A., Defeo-Jones,D., Boyer,M., Martinez,D., Kiefer,D., Vuocolo,G., Wolfe,A., and Socher,S.H. (1987) *Cell*, **50**, 155.
16. Levin,S. and Hahn,T. (1981) *Clin. Exp. Immunol.*, **46**, 475.
17. Shiozawa,S., Yoshikawa,N., Iijima,K., and Negishi,K. (1988) *Clin. Exp. Immunol.*, **73**, 366.
18. Schaffer,N., Grau,G.E., Hedberg,K., Davachi,F., Lyamba,B., Hightower,A.W., Breman,J.G., and Nguyen-Dinh,P. (1991) *J. Infect. Dis.*, **163**, 96.
19. Grau,G.E., Kindler,V., Piguet,P.F., Lambert,P.H., and Vassali,P. (1988) *J. Exp. Med.*, **168**, 1499.
20. Grau,G.E., Heremans,H., Piguet,P.F., Pointaire,P., Lambert,P.H., Billiau,A., and Vassali,P. (1989) *Proc. Natl. Acad. Sci. USA*, **86**, 5572.
21. Mossman,T.R. and Coffman,R.L. (1989) *Annu. Rev. Immunol.*, **7**, 145.
22. Hamid,Q., Azzawi,M., Ying,S., Moqbel,R., Wardlaw,A.J., Corrigan,C.J., Bradley,B., Durham,S.R., Collins,J.V., Jeffery,P.K., Quint,D.J., and Kay,A.B. (1991) *J. Clin. Invest.*, **87**, 1541.
23. Kay,A.B., Ying,S., Varney,V., Gaga,M., Durham,S.R., Moqbel,R., Wardlaw, A.J., and Hamid,Q. (1991) *J. Exp. Med.*, **173**, 775.
24. Sher,A. and Coffman,R.L. (1992) *Annu. Rev. Immunol.*, **10**, 385.
25. Heinzel,F.P., Sadick,M.D., Mutha,S.S., and Locksley,R.M. (1991) *Proc. Natl. Acad. Sci. USA*, **88**, 7011.

26. Boom,W.H., Liebster,L., Abbas,A.K., and Titus,R.G. (1990) *Infect. Immun.*, **58**, 3863.
27. Scott,P., Natovitz,P., Coffman,R.L., Pearce,E., and Sher,A. (1988) *J. Exp. Med.*, **168**, 1675.
28. Yamamura,M., Uyemura,K., Deans,R.J., Weinberg,K., Rea,T.H., Bloom,B.R., and Modlin,R.L. (1991) *Science*, **254**, 277.
29. Salgame,P., Abrams,J.S., Clayberger,C., Goldstein,H., Convit,J., Modlin,R.L., and Bloom,B. (1991) *Science*, **254**, 279.
30. Hanafusa,T., Pujol-Borrell,R., Chiovato,L., Russell,R.C.G., Doniach,D., and Bottazzo,G.F. (1983) *Lancet*, **ii**, 1111.
31. Bottazzo,G.F., Pujol-Borrell,R., Hanafusa,T., and Feldmann,M. (1983) *Lancet*, **ii**, 1115.
32. Todd,I., Pujol-Borrell,R., Abdul-Karim,B.A.S., Hammond,L.J., Feldmann,M., and Bottazzo,G.F. (1987) *Clin. Exp. Immunol.*, **69**, 532.
33. Pujol-Borrell,R., Todd,I., Doshi,M., Gray,D., Feldmann,M., and Bottazzo,G.F. (1986) *Clin. Exp. Immunol.*, **65**, 128.
34. Londei,M., Bottazzo,G.F., and Feldmann,M.N. (1985) *Science*, **228**, 85.
35. Todd,I., Pujol-Borrell,R., Hammond,L.J., and Bottazzo,G.F. (1985) *Clin. Exp. Immunol.*, **61**, 265.
36. Klein,B., Zhang,X.G., Jourdan,M., Content,J., Houssiau,F., Aarden,L., Piechaczyk,M., and Bataille,R. (1989) *Blood*, **73**, 517.
37. Arima,N., Daitoku,Y., Yamamoto,Y., Fujimoto,K., Ohgaki,S., Kojima,K., Fukumori,J., Matsushita,K., Tanaka,H., and Onoue,K. (1987) *J. Immunol.*, **138**, 3069.
38. Cozzolino,F., Rubartelli,A., Aldinucci,D., Sitia,R., Torcia,M., Shaw,A.R., and Di Guglielmo,R. (1989) *Proc. Natl. Acad. Sci. USA*, **86**, 2369.
39. Merz,H., Houssiau,F.A., Orscheschek,K., Renauld,J.C., Fliedner,A., Herin,M., Noel,H., Kadin,M., Mueller-Hermelink,H.K., Van Snick,J., and Feller,A.C. (1991) *Blood*, **78**, 1311.
40. Ymer,S., Tucker,Q.J., Sanderson,C.J., Hapel,A.J., Campbell,H.D., and Young,J.G. (1985) *Nature*, **317**, 255.
41. Arya,S.K. and Gallo,R.C. (1987) *Lymphokines*, **13**, 35.
42. Mitelman,F. (1985) In *Progress and topics in cytogenetics* (ed. A.A.Sanberg). A.R.Liss, New York. Vol. 5, p. 107.
43. Yoshida,H., Hayashi,S.-I., Kunisada,T., Ogawa,M., Nishikawa,S., Okamura,H., Sudo,T., Shultz,L.D., and Nishikawa,S.-I. (1990) *Nature*, **345**, 442.
44. Paul,W.E. (1992) *Nature*, **357**, 16.
45. Stewart,C.L., Kaspar,P., Brunet,L.J., Bhatt,H., Gadi,H., Köntgen,F., and Abbondanzo,S.J. (1992) *Nature*, **359**, 76.
46. Feldmann,M., Brennan,F., and Maini,R. (1993) In *Clinical applications of cytokines: role in pathogenesis and therapy* (ed. J.J.Oppenheim, J.Rossio, and A.Gearing), in press.
47. Granowitz,E.V., Clark,B.D., Vannier,E., Callahan,M.V., and Dinarello,C.A. (1992) *Blood*, **79**, 2356.
48. Granowitz,E.V., Vannier,E., Poutsiaka,D.D., and Dinarello,C.A. (1992) *Blood*, **79**, 2364.
49. Feldman,M. (1991) *Eur. Cytokine Netw.*, **2**, 5.
50. Moore,M.A. (1991) *Annu. Rev. Immunol.*, **9**, 159.
51. Donahue,R.E., Wang,E.A., Stone,D.K., Kaman,R., Wong,G.G., Sehgal,P.K., Nathan,D.G., and Clark,S.C. (1986) *Nature*, **321**, 872.
52. Nienhuis,A.W., Donahue,R.E., Karlsson,S., Clark,S.C., Agricola,B., Antinoff,N., Pierce,J.E., Turner,P., Anderson,W.F., and Nathan,D.G. (1987) *J. Clin. Invest.*, **80**, 573.

53. Welte,K., Bonilla,M.A., Gillio,A.P., Boone,T.C., Potter,G.K., Gabrilove,J.L., Moore,M.A.S., O'Reilly,R.J., and Souza,L.M. (1987) *J. Exp. Med.*, **165**, 941.
54. Gorin,N.C. (ed.) (1992) *Malgramostim GM-CSF: possibilities and perspectives.* Royal Soc. Med. Publications Ltd, London and New York.
55. Maroun,J.A. and Buskard,N.A. (eds) (1992) *Colony-stimulating factors in clinical practice.* Royal Soc. Med. Publications Ltd, London and New York.
56. Grimm,E.A., Mazumder,A., Zhang,H.Z., and Rosenberg,S.A. (1982) *J. Exp. Med.*, **155**, 1823.
57. Mule,J.J., Shu,S., Schwarz,S.L., and Rosenberg,S.A. (1984) *Science*, **225**, 1487.
58. Rosenberg,S.A., Lotze,M.T., Muul,L.M., Leitman,S., Chang,A.E., Ettinghausen,S.E., Matory,Y.L., Skibber,J.M., Shiloni,E., Vetto,J.T., Seipp,C.A., Simpson,C., and Reichert,C. (1985) *N. Engl. J. Med.*, **313**, 1485.
59. Nathan,C.F., Horowitz,C.R., De la Harpe,J.D., Vadhan-Raj,S., Sherwin,S.A., Oettgen,H.F., and Krown,S.E. (1985) *Proc. Natl. Acad. Sci. USA*, **82**, 8686.
60. Thompson,J.A. and Fefer,A. (1987) *Cancer*, **59**, 605.
61. Volberding,P.A., Mitsuyasu,R.T., Golando,J.P., and Spiegel,R.J. (1987) *Cancer*, **59**, 620.
62. Talpaz,M., Kantarjian,H.M., McCredie,K.B., Keating,M.J., Trujillo,J., and Gutterman,J. (1987) *Blood*, **69**, 1280.
63. Castanzi,J.J., Cooper,M.R., Scarffe,J.H. Ozer,H., Grubbs,S.S. Ferraresi,R.W., Pollard,R.B., and Spiegel,R.J. (1985) *J. Clin. Oncol.*, **3**, 654.
64. Lejeune,F. (1992) *Eur. Cytokine Netw.*, **3**, 125.
65. Williams,D.E., Broxmeyer,H.E., Curtis,B.M., Dunn,J., Price,V., Craig,V., March,C.J., Cosmann,D., and Park,L.S. (1990) *Exp. Haematol.*, **18**, 615.
66. Nathan,C.F., Kaplan,G., Levis,W.R., Nusrat,A., Witmer,M.D., Sherwin,S.A., Job,C.K., Horowitz,C.R., Steinmann,R.M., and Cohn,Z.A. (1986) *N. Engl. J. Med.*, **315**, 6.
67. Byrne,G. and Turco,J. (eds) (1988) *Interferon and nonviral pathogens.* Immunology Series, Volume 42, Marcel Dekker, New York.
68. Dinarello,C.A. and Wolff,S.W. (1993) *N. Eng. J. Med.*, **328**, 106.
69. Sher,A., Fiorentino,D., Casper,P., Pearce,E.J., and Mosmann,T.R. (1991) *J. Immunol.*, **147**, 2713.
70. Bock,B.R. and Marsh,J. (eds) (1991) *Clinical applications of TGF-β.* Ciba Foundation Symposium 157. John Wiley and Sons, Chichester.

6

Endpiece: cytokines—the future

Cytokines are polypeptides with powerful and wide-ranging effects on the immune system and beyond. In 20 years they have emerged from being thought to have a restricted role as mediators of cellular immunity, to being known to influence other physiological systems. Thus, they not only activate and amplify cellular responses to antigens but also mediate many responses to stress. Coincident with our appreciation that immune cells are not solely involved with defence against infection has come experimental evidence that cytokines influence many cell types in many organs where they facilitate intercellular communication. As such they are of interest not only to immunologists but also to cell biologists and physiologists concerned with both homeostasis and dysfunction at the cellular and whole-animal level.

Much of what we know about the biological activity of cytokines has come from *in vitro* experiments. It is possible that some of these activities are rarely or never seen *in vivo*. There is a pressing need to understand how and where cytokines work *in vivo*. The physiological importance of cytokines is becoming more evident from experiments in transgenic and gene-deleted (knock-out) mice. These experiments provide fascinating insights and show that we really do not know much of what cytokines do *in vivo* or how they do it.

Immune responses occur primarily in tissues, particularly lymph nodes, where T and B cells are organized into discrete areas in association with antigen-presenting cells. Which cells have receptors for cytokines in normal and diseased tissues? As antibodies to cytokine receptors become available we are able to begin to look at this. Which cells make cytokines and when? Techniques such as *in situ* hybridization provide useful information regarding the spatial and temporal production of cytokines during an immune response. We have little idea about the cytokine concentrations in intercellular spaces or the distance over which a cytokine can act and these issues are of great importance for appreciating the potential a cytokine has for exerting its effects systemically. This in turn is important for our view of regulation of haematopoiesis during stress, cachexia, and so on, where it is envisaged that cytokines produced at a distant site (where?) might influence many body systems.

Gene cloning has provided homogeneous material for biological studies which has been invaluable in delineating the wide variety of activities which most cytokines have. It has also provided material in sufficient quantity to be used for clinical trials, and for crystallization and examination of tertiary structure. In these areas there has been much progress in recent years. We now know that cytokines can positively affect clinical outcome in a variety of diseases and this in itself is a major achievement. Their potential will take some time to realize as studies are needed to define the optimum non-toxic levels. Since it is likely that in many situations 'cocktails' of cytokines may be beneficial, it will take time to assemble the information on these substances separately and together. Interesting further approaches will be to modify cytokines to create new proteins which are active but non-toxic. In diseases where cytokine production seems to be abnormal there will be progress in modifying production by antibodies, soluble receptors, and other inhibitors. Rather than the need to alter cytokine production continuously, it is to be hoped that as we understand more about cytokine networks it may be possible to 'tip the balance' to restore a normal pattern of production with limited intervention.

Although we have recombinant cytokines there is still a need to measure cytokines in biological fluids, *in vitro* and *in vivo*. To effect this there are many immunoassays and bioassays. The choice rests on the question being asked and very often both immunoassay and bioassays are needed to provide useful and complete information. Both types of assay require standardization if results are to be compared within and between laboratories. Human cytokine standards and reference reagents are available and should be incorporated in assays, but a big effort is needed to ensure that their use is adopted and ultimately that the units in which activity is expressed conform to internationally agreed standards.

One of the most rapidly developing areas of cytokine research of recent years has been the cloning of cytokine receptors. The impetus for this has come from industry where knowledge of cytokine receptor structure is invaluable for understanding cytokine action on cells and for attempting to modify such action by creation of antagonists and agonists. Knowledge of cytokine interactions with cytokine receptors, including co-crystallization, will also be invaluable in the process. Also being studied with great fervour is the mechanism of cell signalling by cytokines bound to receptors.

How many cytokines are there? This remains unknown but is likely to be considerably more than those known at present. Ultimately the conclusion of the human genome project will reveal the final number. Why are there so many and why do they have similar activities? It is a general feature of the immune system that there is considerable redundancy and presumably the multiple actions of cytokines reflects a failsafe mechanism to ensure that the immune response occurs.

In this book I have described the structure and function of some of the cytokines. The relative importance of these different proteins will alter as research continues. New cytokines will achieve a significance as new discoveries are made, and then find a natural equilibrium in scientific vocabulary and thought.

The last decade has seen a remarkable change in our perception of these fascinating proteins. The future will undoubtedly prove equally fascinating as more is discovered. There is still much to be learned about the biology and biochemistry of cytokines and their receptors.

Glossary

Autocrine: referring to the way in which a cell can produce a factor which acts on itself (cf. paracrine).

Bioassay: a method for measuring molecules such as cytokines via their physiological actions on cells or living creatures.

Cachexia: weight loss and wasting often seen in individuals carrying tumours.

CD molecules: a system of nomenclature for leucocyte surface molecules, including:

CD2, present on T cells and involved in antigen non-specific cell activation;

CD3, present on T cells associated with the antigen receptor and involved in antigen-specific cell activation;

CD4, present primarily on helper T cells and involved in class-II-restricted interactions;

CD8, present primarily on cytotoxic T cells and involved in class-I-restricted interactions;

CD11/CD18, adhesion molecules expressed on all leucocytes;

CD16, Fc IgG receptor present on natural killer cells and neutrophils;

CD23, the low affinity Fcε receptor;

CD25, present on antigen-activated T and B cells acting as a receptor for IL-2;

CD56, present on natural killer cells;

cDNA: DNA formed by reverse transcription of messenger (m) RNA.

cDNA library: a set of DNA fragments prepared on mRNA templates from a particular cell type. The fragments are expanded by gene cloning.

Chemokines: chemotactic cytokine family.

Colony stimulating factors: a group of molecules which promote division and differentiation of particular lineages of haematopoietic cells.

Delayed type hypersensitivity: a measure of helper T cell reactivity to a particular antigen, detected as a hypersensitivity reaction developing over 24–72 h following application of the antigen to the skin.

Domain: a globular region of folded polypeptide. Antigen receptors and MHC molecules are formed into domains.

Edman Degradation: technique for analysing the amino acid residue sequence of a peptide.

Endotoxin: a component of Gram negative bacterial cell walls (lipopoly-saccharide) which can induce B cell mitogenesis, macrophage activation, complement activation and vascular shock.

Exon: gene segment encoding protein.

Glycosylation: the process of adding carbohydrate groups.

Haemopoiesis: the process of replenishing circulating erythrocytes and leucocytes from stem cells in the fetal liver or bone marrow.

Homology: similar in structure.

Interferons: a group of glycoproteins which act on cells to interfere with viral replication. They also have many other physiological and immunomodulatory effects.

Interleukins: a group of molecules involved in signalling between leucocytes, and other cells in the body.

Introns: gene segments between exons not encoding protein.

Lymphokines: a group of cytokines produced by lymphocytes or lymphoblastoid cells.

Monokines: a group of cytokines made by monocytes or macrophages.

Open reading frame: a stretch of DNA may be read in one of three frames depending on the alignment of the codons. An open reading frame is the one which does not contain stop codons.

Paracrine: acting on other cells (cf. autocrine).

Pleiotropy: the product of a single gene being able to produce two or more effects.

Progenitor cell: cell (often a stem cell) which can give rise to mature cells.

Retrovirus: a group of viruses which have RNA as their genetic material, but which reverse transcribe this into DNA which may become integrated into the host cell nuclear DNA.

Signal sequence: a short stretch of amino acids at the amino-terminus of a polypeptide which directs the translation of the remainder of the polypeptide across the membrane of the endoplasmic reticulum. It is cleaved from the mature protein.

Site-directed mutagenesis: a technique for identifying the active amino acid residues in a ligand–receptor interaction, by selectively changing individual residues and looking for alterations in the function of the protein.

Stem cells: precursor cells which undergo division and give rise to the various lineages of differentiated haematopoietic cells.

Synergy: acting or working together.

Transformed cell: a cell which can give rise to a tumour and which has lost normal growth control.

Transgenic: refers to an animal in which genes from another species have been transplanted.

Index